WAKE UP

YOUR BODY + MIND AFTER 50!

By
MALIN SVENSSON

Disclaimer

The Nordic Body programs in this book offer information for exercising and eating designed for educational purposes only. You should not rely on the information presented as a substitute for, nor does it replace, professional medical advice, diagnosis, or treatment. If you have any concerns or questions about your health, you should always consult a physician or other healthcare provider before starting any exercise and eating programs. Do not disregard, avoid, or delay obtaining medical or health-related advice from your healthcare professional because of something you may have read in any Nordic Body programs. The use of any information provided in the Nordic Body programs is solely at your own risk. No assurance can be given that the advice for exercising and eating contained in the Nordic Body programs will always include the most recent findings and developments with respect to the material.

Dedication

In memory of my wonderful parents, who always believed I could do anything I set my mind to. Thank you, Mamma, and Pappa for teaching me how to live a fun, healthy, and fulfilling life!

Table of Contents

Introduction

Academy Award-winning Actress Olympia Dukakis said my fitness training was innate. English is not my native language, Swedish is, so the word "innate" was not in my vocabulary. She explained her feelings about my work further. "Malin, it is the way you work out with the maturing population that comes so naturally to you - it's like you were born with that skill."

I was simply doing what I felt best served with my lifetime of experiences, and I saw she was right. Going down memory lane, I can see how my whole life I have been gearing up to fulfill my passion - to inspire the 50+ crowd to get a strong body and mind to live a fun, healthy, and fulfilling life.

I had my first view of the aging body with my favorite grandmother, Farmor Lowa, whom I deeply loved and cared for. She was the sweetest and most loving person I have ever known - she could never harm a fly. No matter what time of the day or night you decided to visit her, she would always be happy to see you. She would give you that warm hug with an extremely strong hand patting your behind. It was so powerful that you had to hold your breath for a few seconds. Though she was petite, she was super strong - she did not even know her own strength. I never had the heart to tell her that those hands of hers were so darn strong they actually stung. When she had an unfortunate accident and hurt her arm, I helped her practice the rehab exercises prescribed by the physical therapist. My job was to throw a tennis ball to her that she was supposed to catch with one hand. I was in my early teens and quite the athlete. After a while I got a little bit frustrated with her not being able to catch the ball each time. "Why can't you catch the ball?" I asked.

She stopped and gave me a firm answer - as firm as her hand. "Malin, when you are 80 years old, I'm going to look down from Heaven and see how well you can catch a ball with one hand!"

We both laughed so hard. To this day that answer still cracks me up. It definitely gave the youthful and ignorant me something to think about. **Aging Awareness!**

Every summer job I had during the school years, I would work at nursing homes and hospitals for the elderly, and sometimes at mental illnesses facilities. Seeing how some of the jaded nurses did everything the same way day in and day out made me feel sad for the patients. The patients got excellent care, but the environment itself lacked joy. I wanted to bring something different to my workplace. I was determined to inspire everyone around me, including myself, to get and stay strong in our bodies and minds to stay independent as we age so we can live at home instead of at a nursing home.

Since I just worked there temporarily in the summertime, I had tons of energy, so I started to arrange masquerades, barbeques, and entertainment. Seeing the joy, excitement, and curiosity among patients brought a big smile to all of us. It is a feeling that has stayed with me for all these years. **Alive and Awake Aging!**

When my dad turned 50, I had another age awareness experience. One of the presents he received was a painting that depicted a person going through life from birth to death. There was an arch with steps, each one illustrating a new decade. At the top step you were 50 years old and from then on it was all downhill. Even though I was just 12 years old, the gravity of this image had a huge impact on me. I thought it was the most depressing painting I had ever seen. Every time I looked at that arch, I knew I was not going to live *that* life! I was going to live life like an ascending staircase! **Active and Ageless Aging!**

When I first started out as a personal fitness trainer, I focused mainly on strengthening the physical body. After experiencing both my parents' dementia, I was convinced that we need to take care of our brain and our mind just as much as our physical body to live a long life with quality. We just live once! And it's short. Let's make the most out of it. Let's live life to its fullest! Turning 50 is a milestone in life. Some people celebrate this occasion, and others let it quietly pass on by. Some people look at life as an arch and feel they are at the top when they hit 50. From then on, it's all downhill. Some people view life as an ascending staircase with each step as a new chapter in their life. Which person are you and if you are looking at life as downhill, perhaps we can change your mind and body together.

How about this perspective - Age 50 is only halfway up. From then on, you have all the mistakes, experiences, and lessons behind you to inform you how to have the best life ahead of you. What do you think? If you didn't have the curiosity about life before, and you are turning to me to do better for the next 50, you are in the right place.

Since 1992, I've specialized in working with the 50+ population as a personal fitness trainer. I know what does and doesn't work to age with confidence. This book is based on my philosophy about how to best take care of your health – all aspects of health – physical, mental, emotional, spiritual, and social. Together we will get your body, mind, and brain stronger and healthier. During this journey, don't be surprised if you change the way you think about what you are capable of doing at your age and beyond.

With age we get wiser. The elderly in a tribe used to be the person you'd listen to for advice. Today aging is perceived as being weak instead of respected. Let's disrupt aging by making ourselves as strong as we can with both body and mind to have the best decades to come. Let's convince the younger generation they can still count on us. I challenged one of my wonderful nieces in her twenties, almost half my age, to race the stairs to the 5th floor. She always took the elevator. I beat her even though she was a runner. Now she only takes the stairs. Just because we are older doesn't mean we are held back. We can still be influential to people younger than us, give advice and be a role model.

Olympia Dukakis also inspired me to teach other fitness professionals my system. Why? When she was out here in Los Angeles, she told me she wished I had

Nordic Body Instructors in New York. Before Olympia Dukakis pursued a successful acting career, she was a physical therapist. When she suggested I start teaching other fitness professionals my system, I knew it came from her professional advice as a PT and I felt very honored. Though it would take many years before I finished my Nordic Body Academy Certificate Program for Fitness Professionals, she was the initiator of the idea. She would always tell me how different my workouts were and how I prepared for them like she prepared for an acting role – meticulously.

My clients keep inspiring me. During the Corona Virus Pandemic, Tony Award Winning Actress (and one of the stars of the hit Netflix show *Grace and Frankie*) Lily Tomlin asked me if we could continue working out online. Even though I have worked with the 50+ since 1992, and I am the first one to say anything is possible at any age, I still had a preconceived idea that people in their 80's and up would not be interested in online training. Wrong! Lily made it possible for me to keep a thriving fitness business online during and after the pandemic. She helped expand my own mindset about training my clients online.

The day Fitness Guru, Activist and Academy Award Winning Actress Jane Fonda walked up to me in a gym and asked if I could work her out was the ultimate confirmation my fitness training system was unique. Jane Fonda hiring me as her workout trainer was akin to the Dali Lama hiring a spiritual teacher. To this day, I am extremely honored and proud to be Jane Fonda's "workout trainer" (as she calls me). At the same time, I knew her acknowledgment was my cue to bring my Nordic Body System to a bigger audience.

In fact, while reading Jane Fonda's book "Prime Time," I jumped at least twice because she mentioned two concepts that I have practiced all my life. I had never heard anyone verbalize them. The first concept was about the disempowering traditional arch of life (you're at the top when you're 50) versus the empowering way of aging like a staircase where you continue to evolve and explore life. Exactly like the "a-ha" moment I experienced as a pre-teenager from observing the depressing painting my dad received on his 50th birthday. The second concept is her

"Review of Life." Reading her book and knowing her, I had a moment of clarity, because I had been doing this life assessment all my life, but I call it the "Map of Your Life." I felt even more connected to her. The way she chooses to age with passion and purpose is incredibly inspirational and in alignment with what I have to bring to the world as a wellness expert.

This book is about disrupting aging - I believe we are all ageless. In Chapter One, *Successful Aging,* you will be even more convinced that age is just a number. It doesn't define you. This book can be used by any age, but it has mainly been written for anyone close to age 50 or past 50 and beyond. Though the age range is huge, you will definitely relate to all parts of this book and any specific issue you are dealing with as you are aging. Think about this book as a journey I am leading you through. The goal is to have everything absorbed within three months. You can do one chapter a week or read one chapter a day or finish it all in one weekend. Chapter Two helps you *Awaken Your Mind for Success* and can be applied to any goals and dreams you would like to reach. This chapter is a must-read. This is where most workout programs fail because you haven't set up the commitment in your subconscious first.

The next seven chapters (3 to 9) are the essence of the book. You'll explore different and new ways to move your body, making sure it is pain-free, doing it correctly to stay injury free while getting your muscles, bones, and heart strong, plus improving the flexibility and mobility of the muscles and joints. Some of the instructions are available on videos as well at https://nordicbody.com/wakeup. We make it easy to fulfill your goals by offering different ways to learn.

Chapter Ten *Feed Your Body and Brain* guides you through unique ways of thinking when you choose what foods to put into your mouth. Chapter Eleven shows the obstacles that could arise along your journey and how to deal with them with *Your Success Team,* another key ingredient to succeed.

Chapter Twelve is what actually inspired me the most to write this book. When you have a strong body and mind, *Anything is Possible at Any Age.* I know it is cliché to say you will be transformed, but it is true - at that point in the book you will feel you have so much confidence, freedom, and clarity that anything is possible. Anecdotes of five people's stories of reinventing themselves at any decade from 50-90 will pop up here and there throughout the book to inspire you and realize that "yes, I can do that too."

Writing this book, doing speaking engagements and offering walking and strength training programs online and in person are all part of my greater mission to spread the motivational message to the 50+ population worldwide: "Be your strongest in both your body and your mind to live a fun, healthy and fulfilling life."

"Aging is not lost youth but a new stage
of opportunity and strength."

~**Betty Friedan**

CHAPTER 1:

Successful Aging

How many of you have heard that age is just a chronological number? How many of you believe that? I do. I have worked out people in their 20's who are in bad shape and trained people in their 70's who are in great shape. So yes, our age just informs us how many years we have been on this planet. It doesn't dictate who you are, how young you are at heart, or your attitude towards life. However, as we age, the body - your machine- will experience more wear and tear. That is simply a practical truth. How do we deal with that? We wake up our bodies and minds. Some live in denial, and others rise up to the occasion to protect their body for a longer, happier life. If you are at a place in your life where aspects of your body are holding you back, no matter what age, the time has come to make a change. If you are here with me now reading, you, or someone who loves you, wants that change.

We all deal with age differently. Some brag about their age, some lie about their age, and some refuse to say their age. I say EMBRACE YOUR AGE. Maybe it's easy for me to say that because I had a big party to celebrate turning 50. For others it may be a horrible thought to have the first half of their life passed by. What happened? How did I end up here? A lot of us wake up at 50, 60, 70, 80 and ask ourselves that question which I see as a springboard to take action to build your body and mind so you can live in an extraordinary way for the rest of your life. I think we all can agree that good health can give us quality of life, right?

Excuses in Your Way

Has an unexpected incident, like a fall, for example, suddenly made you feel 20 years **older**? I bet it scared you and brought up uncomfortable feelings about your body and aging. The good news is you don't have to be scared because we have solutions to take a wakeup call as a springboard to stay consistently in shape as you are aging. You can be ready in the future to combat any obstacles that come your way.

Let's look at a variety of great excuses that keep people from exercising and changing bad habits to good healthy ones. You may know someone who lived to be 100 years young without exercising or eating nutritiously. Is that really going to be your argument for not moving your body or eating healthy? Are you really going to use that as an excuse for not exercising? Are you really going to take that risk?

You may have tried exercising in the past without any results. "I've tried it and it didn't work for me." Though I am sorry to hear that, I am also curious to find out why it didn't work. What did you do for exercise? How long did you keep up that routine? Did you change your eating habits? Having worked with the 50+ for 28 years and seeing great results with my clients, I want you to give it a new shot. If you follow the guidelines in this book, I promise you will not be disappointed.

You may say, "Look at athletes - they are injured all the time. Exercising must be bad. I don't want to get injured." True, athletes very often get injured. Then they get the best treatment to get back out there to compete again. BUT there is a reason for athletes hurting themselves a lot. They constantly push their bodies past its limits. We are NOT going to do that here. I'm going to give you instructions on how to operate and manage your body to stay strong and injury-free as long as possible. We all know that if we read instructions on how to care for a certain machine or piece of equipment, it will last much longer, right?

Take your car for example. I bet you sometimes take better care of your car than your body. They both have batteries (your heart), they both need to be oiled (your joints need to be oiled), they both need to get realigned (muscles and joints) from time to time, and sometimes the wear and tear is so severe that some parts have to be replaced. Luckily, today's technology is so amazing that many of our body parts can be replaced, but don't rely on that fact. With surgeries come risks, so take care of your current parts as well as possible to avoid surgery - make that the last option. (That's just my opinion.) Do you have aches and pains that prevent you from exercising? It can be a catch 22. If you exercise, you hurt. If you don't exercise, you will lose strength in both muscles and bones, which will lead to other pain. Some people "accept" their aches and pains while other people do tons of research by asking friends for medical referrals to find solutions. Never give up. There is always a better solution than not doing anything.

Listen to Your Body

Are you alive and awakened, or do you walk around like a zombie through this precious life of yours? Wake up. Many people cut off the communication between their heads and their bodies. Then one day when an ache appears, it is the biggest surprise ever. Why is that hurting? What happened? What did I do? Now the body has finally gotten your attention. The body is so amazing - it has pain receptors telling us that something is not ok. Some of us have higher pain thresholds than others. Regardless of your tolerance for pain, pay attention to it. The worst thing you can do is to ignore it. Time may heal it, but time may also make it worse if you keep repeating things that resulted in the ache. It may be an old, untreated injury gradually preventing you from doing certain physical activities like long hikes. That's what happened to me in my early 40's. An old ankle injury in my teens caught up to me in my early 40's. As a teenager I was competing and training at a high level (one of Sweden's top five female runners in the mid 70's). Two times I twisted my right ankle severely. The ligaments were so stretched out that they never retracted to the length that would keep my ankle stable. When you're younger the body heals faster, however the location of an injury will always remain your weak link. Luckily, I was introduced to NASM (National Academy of Sports Medicine), became NASM

Certified, and learned how to do trigger release. Within two weeks, I could finally sleep at night without waking up with excruciating pain in my right ankle. In Chapter Five, I will share how you can use trigger release to deal with aches and pains.

If Not Now, When?

Living in Los Angeles, I see all the time how the fast-paced city can be cruel to the elderly. Isn't it sad to see a person with a cane or a limp rushing as fast as they can to make the light and still not be able to do it? I'm sure we see people around us all the time **that we don't want to end up like when we grow older**. NOW is the perfect time for you to do something about it. Change your future right here, right now. This is your chance to improve your health - your body and mind. Investment into your health is the best investment there is. If not now, then when? What is the alternative? You're at the top of your game in your mid-twenties - you are your strongest in both muscle strength and bone strength. Nevertheless, your strength also starts to decline in this decade if you don't do maintenance. This is a piece of knowledge you may want to pass on to your kids and grandkids to motivate them to start early.

When you do not take care of your health here are just a few examples of what happens to your body:

- Your muscles will atrophy, and you will not only find yourself with flabby muscles, but also not having the strength to do daily activities that you now take for granted.
- With weaker muscles, your bones will also weaken, so if you were to fall, you will be more prone to fractures.
- Your heart will be less proficient in pumping out blood (transporting oxygen) to all the working organs and muscles. Oxygen is life! Without oxygen nothing will work. That goes for your brain as well.

Even if you are the smartest person on earth and you know all the benefits from taking care of your health, you still may not take action. If you are not familiar with all the life-changing benefits from exercising, you can look them up in different chapters in this book. For example, in Chapter Four, I will give you the benefits from leading an active lifestyle like taking the stairs instead of the escalator. In Chapter Seven, I will give you the benefits from strength training like sitting down and standing up from a chair. In Chapter Eight the benefits from cardiovascular training like walking and in Chapter Nine the benefits from stretching to avoid feeling stiffness.

Moving Past the Top Three Excuses

Lack of **motivation, time,** and **knowledge** are the top three excuses we use to not commit to taking care of our health - especially exercising. Change starts with awareness of what we need to change before we can change it. Do you ever use any of the three excuses? Which one do you use the most? Can you relate to them? Be truthful – it's the only way to make progress.

1. Motivation

Lacking motivation is the number one excuse. I hear about it all the time. If we don't feel motivated to do something, we most likely won't do it. Throughout the book, you will get more and more motivated. There are even some places where we work on your big "why" to be able to stick to a healthy routine. At the end of this chapter, the *Reality Check* assignment including the *Body Map* will increase your awareness. This in itself can act as a motivation. My main motivation to take care of my health is you. I want to be a role model for you to inspire you to take care of your health after 50 to live a fun, healthy and fulfilling life.

Let's make a list of fun, healthy and fulfilling ideas that can motivate YOU:

1. Have enough strength to play with my kids, grandkids, nieces, and nephews.

2. Be able to go on romantic walks with my loved one.

3. Get ready for an event like a reunion, wedding, birthday.

4. Have better stamina and energy to socialize more.

5. Make the dream trip and adventure of my life.

6. _____

7. _____

8. _____

9. _____

10. _____

How do people age successfully? Who is your role model when it comes to aging? Look at that person's life and see what they have done and what they are doing. Maybe you can even ask them, how do they stay motivated to exercise? Typically, people love to talk about their successes. You just need to ask.

My role model is one of my clients - Jane Fonda. I'm sure many of you agree with me that she is aging very gracefully. At age 82, she is still committed to taking care of her health, working out, eating healthy and having a huge desire and purpose to make a difference in the world. As we all know she's a fitness guru and has taken care of her health all her adult life. However, I believe it's never too late to start working out at any age. Studies show all the time the benefits of even people at age 90 being able to build muscles to get stronger. At the end of this book, I have interviewed my 98-year-old client, Betty Dasteel, who says that she has gotten stronger since we started to work out four years ago. Her advice to all of us is, "Keep moving your body."

2. Time

Number two excuse: "I have no time to work out." How do we find time to take care of our health? I always say, "To experience something you have to make space for it." It's about prioritizing but it is also about changing habits, which is where we encounter resistance. It's important to see the bigger picture and then break down the resistance with small actions. How will you feel or look one year from now? How are you living your life differently? What you do now has to be different if you want to see a change in yourself in the near future. If you keep doing the same thing you will end up with the same result. Let's start small and free up 15 minutes of your time. Look at your schedule and write down the times you have 15 minutes or more to invest daily into your future health. Those sacred 15 minutes will be allocated to movement and taking care of your health. Fifteen minutes? Will that really do something? Yes, it will set you up for victory to start a good habit of moving your body 15 minutes daily compared to now, which may be 0 minutes a day. Are you with me?

FINDING 15 MINUTES DAILY:

Monday: _____

Tuesday: _____

Wednesday: _____

Thursday: _____

Friday: _____

Saturday: _____

Sunday: _____

A lot of people that are motivated right now want immediate results and they give their best for two weeks by working out and eating super healthy every day. That's too dramatic. It's a shock to the body. It won't last. You'll end up thinking every moment about food you can't have, and your body will feel really sore after all the intense workouts because the body hasn't worked out like that in years. You have to make small changes that will last more than two weeks. Take small steps and then add on one more gradually until every new healthy habit feels like it's naturally part of your lifestyle. Making YOU the priority can be difficult especially if you're used to prioritizing other people like your kids, your parents, your loved one, etc. Schedule time for YOU. Make a workout appointment for you. If you're not healthy, you will not be able to take care of other people that need you. To hire a fitness trainer is another solution to prioritize you and your time. If the budget doesn't allow it, ask a dependable and likeminded friend to be your fitness buddy and start walking together instead of getting together for coffee and catching up - or combine it. You can also visit our website https://nordicbody.com/ to see what online or live options we can offer that work for you. It all boils down to being held accountable.

3. Knowledge

The third excuse to not commit to taking care of your health is not knowing what to do. Search no further - you are holding the book that will give you knowledge and instructions step by step on what to do and how to do it to take care of your health after age 50. After finishing this book, you will have a well-rounded knowledge and support from me to succeed with a healthy mind and body. You can join me at my live classes, workshops, and retreats. If the live locations do not work for you, you can join me online. I'm committed to help you - this is one of my missions and passions in life. To dive into working out at this age can be scary. If we don't exercise correctly, we may end up getting injured and that will bring everything to a stop. When we get sick or injured and we try to return to working out, we need to restart with caution and not where we left off. The same thing applies if you haven't worked out in 20-30 years. You can't just pick up where you left off. Your body is different, and you need to honor it and respect it instead of getting frustrated and quitting. After the first couple of workouts, it's better to feel that it was easy, and you may not even be sore (instead of being so sore you can barely take a step). There may be madness to my method, but it works. At one retreat, a woman complained about her right knee. As she did an exercise, her joints were not lined up, so I tried to have her understand how everything has to be stacked on top of each other to work optimally. I started from the ankle and asked her to stack the knee over the ankle then I added knee and hip. Next time she moved the knee was pain-free. Yay!

Where are You in the Circle of Life?

No matter what age you are, it is never too late to be aware that many of our excuses come from fear of what is happening to our bodies as we age. At some point we seem to have forgotten how to move and explore our body. "What happened to that fearless kid on the playground?" fuels the next question: "Why do I feel fear and insecure moving my body now?" I had a client participating at one of my retreats. She used to feel fear moving her body and had many excuses of why she didn't start addressing this fear earlier in life. We worked on her confidence and it sure made a huge difference in her life. She was just turning 60 and her biggest goal was to feel more secure as she walked and moved her body. The motivation emerged, she made time to work out, plus she got the knowledge from me how to overcome the fear. Within a year she was doing a 5k charity walk over an inclined bridge. It was a challenge she had set up in her mind to do and she followed through. What an accomplishment! I'm so proud of her. In the beginning, she just told a few close friends, but as she felt more and more confident of her being able to do it, she began to share with other people as well. You bet she inspired everyone around her.

At some of my workshops and retreats, I tap my clients back into their bodies by reminding them of different development stages of life. I show the journey of what stereotypically happens from the time we are born to the time we die. I call it the *Circle of Life* and as I'm demonstrating the various stages of movement in life, I ask the audience to observe, "What stage are you in your life?" "How did you get here?" "What's your journey?" It's quite an eye-opener to a lot of people who have not been in tune with their gradual physical changes. Unless you have an acute injury, the changes can be so small that we don't notice them until one day we are in front of the mirror seeing our hunched over posture and wondering how did that happen?

The *Circle of Life* demonstration is non-verbal. I start lying down on the floor in a fetal position. From there I incorporate movements that usually happen until the first walking step. Imagine your child, nephew/niece or a friend's child when they were a few months old and how they physically developed:

- Roll over from side to side
- Raise the head and chest when on the tummy.
- Push up on arms when lying on tummy
- Dragging forward by arms and legs on tummy
- Crawling on hands and knees
- Pull up to a standing position.
- Move around holding onto furniture.
- Take first step - usually the weight shifts from side to side ("duck walk") and the concentration of keeping the balance is high

From here on I demonstrate hypothetically what can happen in life to our body.
- Regular walking using the opposite arm and leg creating a natural rotation
- Hop, skip, and jump
- Running to sprinting
- Injury - maybe twisting an ankle or hurting a knee - injury due to inactivity or pushing the body past its limit or due to an unforeseen accident
- The walk is slowed down, maybe even limping and maybe we even stop using the arm swing to just "carry" our arms as we walk with difficulty
- The body starts compensating

- We need to use a cane to be able to move and walk
- We need to use a walker to be able to move and walk
- One day we just can't walk

At some retreats, I actually have people try out the stages from rolling side-to-side on their backs to standing up. Interestingly enough, many people struggle with some of the "infant" movements. If these stages are challenging, you may have challenges walking upright since these movements are building blocks for your body's physical development. In addition, you can see similarities in an infant taking its first step by shifting the weight sideways to better keep the balance, compared to an elderly person who walks side-to-side with a wider stance to feel safer. I see this "duck walk" in a lot in people who are afraid of falling - they don't trust their balance. Try it. Doesn't it feel sturdier to walk side to side with a wider stance (duck walk) then to rotate (opposite arms and leg) as you walk forward? If you already are doing the "duck walk," I hope this will bring some awareness to how you walk and how you should aim to walk. In Chapter Eight, I will show you what a correct walk looks like and exercises you can do to practice correct walk (gait). Walking is a fundamental movement, but if we don't use the correct mechanics, it can gradually lead to injuries. If you have aches and pains when you walk, don't accept it. Take action to do something about it.

In my work as a personal fitness trainer, I specialize in correcting muscular imbalances. Having said that, I want to emphasize that I am not a Physical Therapist. Since 2000, I have been a Certified NASM Personal Fitness Trainer and that is their main approach to strength training - to correct muscular imbalances. It is not bodybuilding and aesthetics. It is getting your body to become more functional to decrease pain and to prevent future injuries so you can live a longer and stronger life with more quality. In Chapter Seven (strength training), you will learn that movement needs to be done correctly to fire the correct muscles before you can load the muscles. We pay attention to the difference in the left side compared to the right side of the body to increase your awareness on how you can improve your body's mechanical system. We get the fire back in your body.

CHECK-IN #1: SUCCESSFUL AGING

Part of helping you increase your awareness of your body is to do a reality check and to create a baseline. Right now, you may feel tons of resistance in doing this action step, but when you can return to this page and jot down new numbers in 4-12 weeks, it will feel great to have established this baseline. Otherwise you won't have anything to compare to. No matter how small the victory, it is worth celebrating. Small changes over time turn into huge changes of feeling better overall. Every new journey starts with one step. Well, this is step one - fill out as much as you can below:

Date___(day)_____(month) _____(year)

1. Create Your Body Map - Mark with an X on areas of your body that hurt.

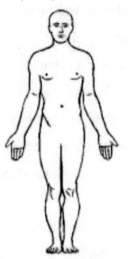 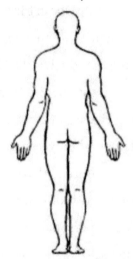

2. Expand on when that area started to hurt and if you know why it started to hurt.

_____

_____

_____

_____

_____

3. How much is the pain? Estimate a number of the subjective pain for each area that hurts. For example, a #10 means that it is so painful you can't move. A #1 means the pain or discomfort you feel is only a reminder that something is not right.

NAME OF THE AREA (for example "knee")   AMOUNT OF PAIN
                                                (for example #5)

_____   #_____

_____   #_____

_____   #_____

_____   #_____

_____   #_____

_____   #_____

_____   #_____

_____   #_____

_____   #_____

As you move your body, your *Body Map* will be part of the puzzle to figure out why your body hurts when you do certain exercises. Always contact a doctor if you are in pain. Do not work out when you're in pain. "No pain no gain" is old school. We don't work through pain; only through fatiguing muscles. Some people can't differentiate between the discomfort one feels from stretching a muscle and fatiguing a muscle, or from an injured muscle. Try to enhance your awareness to distinguish between these three different types of discomfort.

When was the last time you did an annual physical checkup? Fill out as much as you can below. If you don't know the numbers, please book an appointment with your physician. High blood pressure, for example, is called a silent killer. We don't feel the symptoms until a blood vessel bursts and suddenly, we don't get enough oxygen to our heart, brain, muscles etc. Stay smart about the body that carries you through your amazing life and don't have it be cut short by something that could have been prevented.

Annual Physical Exam Results DATE: _____

- Blood Pressure _____

- Cholesterol _____

- Body Weight _____

- Body Height _____

- Body Mass Index _____

Moving your body with freedom is a wonderful feeling. Sometimes we forget how our body used to be able to move. Maybe we are too sedentary, and the body never gets to practice what it was made to do - to move. Maybe we're limited to moving due to injuries and pain. Let's see how your body can and can't move. Do not try any of the movements below if you are not sure you can do it.

Body Movement

- Can you walk up the stairs alternating feet? **yes__ no__**

- Can you walk down the stairs alternating feet? **yes__ no__**

- Can you stand up from and sit down on a chair without help from your hands? **yes__ no__**

- Can you get up and down from the floor without help from any furniture or bars? **yes__ no__**

- How long can you stand on your right leg only without any support? **__ seconds**

- How long can you stand on your left leg only without any support? **__ seconds**

I get tired of hearing excuses about old age. You can feel old at 20 and then come alive again at 60. Bring on the excuses with age, let me debunk them for you, I've heard them all. Let me tell you - I felt old at 22. What happened? I fell in love with Paris and while living in that lovely city, an agent asked me right on the street if I wanted to be a model. I thought, "Hm, this could be a way to make a living while living in Paris." So, I did. After a while, when I realized that a lot of the models were 15-17 years old, I felt old. At the time it felt very real, but now I can look back and chuckle. As I'm getting closer to 60, I feel young and super excited about life and all the treasures it gives me. Luckily, that has been the only time in my life when I have had an age crisis. My advice: don't compare yourself to other people and their accomplishments. Follow YOUR heart and you can never go wrong. I'm here to wake you up both in your body and in your mind. Let's do this together! Let's go!

"You have power over your mind – not outside events.
Realize this, and you will find strength."
~Marcus Aurelius

CHAPTER 2:

Awaken Your Mind for Success!

To WAKE UP your body, we need to WAKE UP your mind! Have you ever said, "On Monday I'm going to start working out" and then you last for one to two weeks before you burn out? The good news is I understand why that is happening and I can help you have consistent success with your body. The issue is you have not primed your mind first. Before we even work with your body - we need to hang out a bit with your mind. I'm a firm believer that if you set up your mind for success, you will have a better chance of succeeding with anything you do in life including taking care of your health. Everything starts with the mind. So, change your thoughts and you will feel motivated to move your body and exercise.

Mindset

The mind is very powerful. Every thought you think affects your body. When was the last time you paid attention to how you feel after a good or bad thought? Have you ever tried to change a negative thought about exercising to a positive one to see if it helped you perform better? It's quite interesting. Try it. When I was a competitive runner in Sweden during my teens, there were many times when the weather was making it more difficult and less enjoyable to train. My running stride felt cumbersome and heavy, as if it was matching the dark mood of the sky and the deep snow. One time I explored, saying to myself "I feel light as a feather." I kept repeating those words over and over again until I actually felt lighter. Wow, what a discovery! Suddenly it was easier to run regardless of the harsh weather. This is a life lesson I have applied to not just exercise, but all areas of my life. Now, don't think I walk around on clouds all the time. I definitely think it's normal and healthy to feel down at times, otherwise we can't enjoy all the ups. It's important to acknowledge that something is bothering you, but it's just as important to figure out how you can change things for the better.

Some people are close-minded. "This is who I am" they believe or, "This is how I was born" or "I can't change." Then there are people that are open-minded and prioritize personal growth regardless of age – they want to stay curious, make changes, and take on new challenges in life that will sustain fulfillment. Which person are you? Fear and perfection prevent some people from making modifications, whereas curiosity and courage encourage people to transform throughout life. Where do you fit in? Our goal together is to have you feel new energy to take charge of your life and keep growing as a human being, and to make a difference for yourself and everyone around you. The mind and body working together naturally takes you in the right direction to achieve that goal.

When we do decide to try something new (a positive change), like start a healthier diet or an exercise regimen, it's very important that we surround ourselves with people that will help us make the new journey easier. Do not hang out with people that will sabotage your new adventure. That is setting yourself up for failure. Sometimes it's even better to not tell those people what you are about to do. Only share it with people that will support you. Think for a moment right now about who could sabotage your efforts and make a mental note to put them in a particular box for now.

Our mindset is crucial. All of us have been there – hearing negative voices and doubting ourselves. Even the most successful people have experienced that. The key is to not fight it. Listen to those voices. They are a part of you. Go deeper and ask productive and quality questions and find out why they (the voices) are cautioning you. Treat each voice as a character in a play. Pretend that you have a whole scene going on in your brain. Sometimes surprising characters (voices) pop up out of the blue trying to tell you something. Listen, understand, and compromise with the specific "character." For example, you are new to working out and you hear an internal voice that says, "Don't exercise, you will get hurt." Listen to the message, understand it and then compromise and say, "What if I start with three simple exercises and make sure I do them correctly to not hurt myself? Will that make you feel better?" If the voice becomes less frantic, then you have negotiated with the fear and won. Every time that voice returns, calm it down and remind it about the compromise.

A sound mind will help you want to invigorate and exercise your body. The critical thing is not to stay in the poisonous environment of negative thoughts – try to snap out of it. Some of those times are easier than other times. If you are medically diagnosed with depression, that is a different scenario and requires a specialized treatment, but you can still try and make a positive change. Life is trial and error. If you didn't try, you wouldn't know about failing. If you don't fail, you haven't stretched to your fullest potential. I listened to an interview one time between Oprah and Steve Harvey. He said to Oprah, "I bet you have failed more times than anyone in this room." Oprah nodded in agreement. You must fail to be successful. If you have, for example, failed to work out before, this is your chance to get it right and make it successful. Developing a healthy mind, and a healthy body work in tandem together

Mental Training

How has your mindset been shaped? What is your mindset based on? My strong mindset today was shaped by my athletic and competitive training in my teens. Here are some of my values that have been part of my mindset since I was eleven.

- Believe in myself.
- Never give up.
- Try my hardest.
- Do my best.

- Not afraid of pushing myself.

- Perseverance.

- Determination.

- Trust my inner wisdom.

Any successful athlete must have both a strong body and mind(set) to win. Mental training can be included in the overall training of an athlete. Can you imagine the concentration, focus, and mindset that are required for a high jumper when the audience goes wild with the bar set on world record high? Or when a tennis player has been playing for hours, tiebreaker after tiebreaker? Or when a golfer is close to winning the British Open? When I went to Sport University in Sweden (G.I.H Orebro), some of my favorite subjects were mental training, anatomy, and biomechanics. The combined education shaped my personal fitness training with emphasis on the importance of having a strong body and a strong mind at any age.

In the mental training course, there was a study of basketball players. They were divided into three groups. One group was told to not train at all during x number of weeks. One group was told to keep on training to make the basket. The third group was told to only sit and mentally envision themselves scoring each time they took a shot at the basket. Guess which group improved the most? Yes, the group that used mental training! The mind cannot differentiate between reality and imagination. One athlete at the 1984 Olympic Games in LA was tested after he had run a race. He was asked to relive (re-run) the race in his mind while he was sitting down connected to machines measuring his blood pressure, heart rate, etc. He used his imagination so well that his blood pressure and heart rate went up as high when he was racing even though he was just sitting thinking about the race. Pretty powerful, huh? Later in this chapter you get to explore some visualization techniques as you meditate to empower your mindset.

Mindfulness

Have you ever been in a zone where the past or future didn't exist - just the present? Consider yourself lucky. That's the goal with mindfulness. To just be in the moment. Some people experience it when they are completely immersed in something so interesting or so intense that the focus must be on the present. I experienced it when I was competing as an 800-meter runner, but also one time when I was swimming with wild dolphins in Hawaii. It was absolutely amazing, yet scary, to feel part of the pod of 20 dolphins swimming with me, around me, and below me. There were four playful dolphins below me, constantly turning over to show me their white bellies. There was one dolphin that never left my side and felt like it was the dolphin from a dream I had many years earlier that resulted in this real dream of swimming with wild dolphins. Needless to say, I was heavily immersed into being a dolphin. Immersed to the point that neither the past nor the future existed. Absolute bliss. The scary part happened when I woke up from this bliss feeling. I must have swum for hours with the dolphins and thought our boat was far, far away. Since I was only snorkeling, I popped up my head, seeing to my relief that I was not that far away from the boat.

Reliving my dolphin experience helped me immensely one time when I was quite nervous during a dental surgery. To practice mindfulness means that you are present and focused on only one thing. Use all your senses to experience it instead of being on autopilot. Look at the trees when you walk, acknowledge the people that you meet, smell the roses you pass by, stop to pet a friendly dog, and listen to the birds sing. Compare talking with someone who is distracted to a person who is fully present when you talk. Quite a difference, right? It feels much better when somebody is really listening to you instead of multi-tasking. Especially if you have something to say that is very important to you. Sometimes you may even choose to not say it because you feel the person is not listening anyway.

Meditation

Mindfulness is being aware of one thing, being fully present. Mindfulness is a form of meditation. You can experience it below in the *Breath and Body Awareness* Meditation. First, let's discover some wonderful, and maybe surprising, benefits from meditation to motivate you to start a daily easy practice. We definitely all need it in this fast-paced society. We need to go inward to feel calmness unless you're relaxing on a deserted island without a worry in your mind.

- Reduces stress and anxiety (source Mayo Clinic)
- Decreases and prevents dementia (source Harvard)
- Help change the plasticity of the brain. (source Sara Lazar, Harvard)

Before it was believed that the brain just kept on losing brain cells as we age, but today there are many studies showing that we can make changes in the brain. We can change, we can learn new things, we can constantly expand and grow as we age.

Three Different Meditations

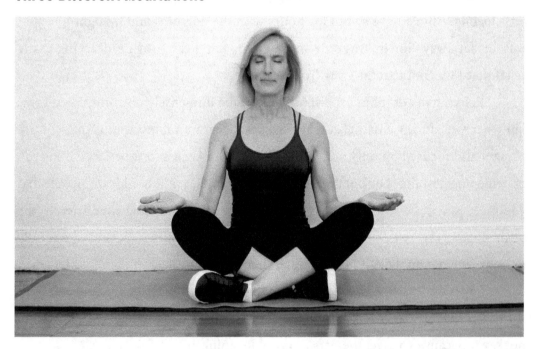

Spiritual Meditation is not for everyone – we all have different tastes and beliefs, but I want to share three different ways that I teach meditation (Awareness, Active, and Spiritual). I hope one or all of them is something you can try out.

1. *Breath & Body Awareness Meditation*

As a personal fitness trainer, I very often take people through a simple mindfulness exercise to calm them down. For example, I start my session with my 98-year-old client with this practice for about 5-10 minutes. As she ages, she finds that things that seemed small 30 years ago can be big and stressful today, so I like to help her find her grounding before we exercise together. If you have a difficult time with the word "meditation," just do this breathing and awareness of your body exercise that I have created. If 5 minutes feels too long, start with one minute. The consistency is more important than the duration.

- Arrange to not be disturbed for your preferred meditation time.
- Set a timer or use a meditation app.
- Light a candle to add to the ambience of peacefulness.
- Sit on the edge of a chair to stay alert - if you have back pain, add back support.
- Keep your feet on the ground and place your hands lightly on your lap.
- Close your eyes.
- Take three deep breaths in and out through the nose.
- Feel how you calm down. Keep breathing slowly and deeply.
- Bring your awareness to your feet. Feel them flat on the floor with all ten toes connected to the ground. Feel grounded and rooted through your feet to Mother Earth.
- Bring your awareness to your spine. Sit nice and tall. Pretend there is a string from the crown of your head that pulls you up to lengthen your spine every time you breathe out. Feel empowered and connected to the sky above you.
- Keep breathing slowly and deeply and feel how you are being pulled in two directions to elongate your whole body. Push down towards the feet and pull up through the crown of your head. Feel awake and alive.

- Bring your awareness to your shoulders. Next time you breathe out pull the shoulders away from your ears and lengthen the neck. Feel the tension in your shoulders melt away.

- Stay with your shoulders. Gently bring the shoulder blades together in the back. Feel the chest opening. Feel the freedom. Feel your heart opening up. Feel the love.

- Stay here a few minutes and repeat to the rhythm of your breath the following two words: Breathe and Be. As you inhale, silently say, "Breathe." As you exhale, silently say, "Be."

- When you are ready to open your eyes, do it only halfway. Open your eyes slowly and softly only halfway. Keep the awareness of your slow and deep breathing.

- Then slowly open up your eyes fully, still staying connected to the slow and deep breathing.

During the day when you ever feel tension or stress return to taking three deep breaths repeating Breathe & Be or any positive affirmations that are meaningful to you.

The *Breath & Body Awareness* meditation is available on audio at https://nordicbody.com/wakeup

2. Active Meditation

Do you recall the story about the Olympic athlete who used his imagination so well that he tricked his mind into believing he was racing again even though he was just sitting on a chair? Now it's your turn to use your power of believing and visualizing. The conscious mind has been conditioned your whole life based on your beliefs, experiences, and habits. The subconscious mind is what we need to tap into to make new lasting changes. It is your guiding system. We need to go deeper than just saying, "Tomorrow I will start eating healthier." We need to use our conscious minds to make a decision on what we want (goal), how we will reach the goal (plan), create action steps, and enter the actions steps into your calendar to make it happen. At the same time, we will get the subconscious mind to visualize the outcome of the goal by use of your imagination. Then your mind thinks that goal is happening right now. Make it as real as possible as you continue to meditate.

1. Place a journal and a pen next to you.

2. Use the *Breath & Body Awareness Meditation* guidelines to get into a good sitting position with good posture.

3. Close your eyes and get ready to use your imagination. Visualize how you will feel when you have reached your goal of Waking Up Your Body + Mind. For example, you are feeling and looking good, strong, and confident. Use all the five senses: sight, hearing, smell, taste, and touch to make it as real as you can. What do you see? How do you feel? What do you hear? What do you smell? How does it feel to touch your body?

4. Now turn that imagination into something that is happening right now. The mind doesn't know the difference between reality and imagination. Make it real for the mind and for you. Believe it is happening right now. You have created a movie. Play that movie on the screen in your mind. Imagine your closed eyes are that screen. The movie is, for example, about you feeling and looking good, strong, and confident.

5. Let the image (the movie) go. Sit and breathe for the remaining time of your meditation. Send the message out into the universe and surrender.

6. Finish the meditation the same gentle way as the *Breath & Body Awareness Meditation*.

Crucial Post Meditation Steps to Reset Your Mind for Success

- Pick up your journal and write down the image of your own personal movie you imagined and all the senses you experienced. Create a vision board that gives you the same wonderful feeling you had during the "movie."

- Create a few action steps that need to happen for this goal of yours to come true. You can complete this as you are reading the book.

- Spend a few minutes a day of looking at your goals on the vision board and the action steps, especially prior to next time you want to do an Active Meditation.

Creating your personal movie of the new healthy you in your subconscious has really primed your mind to be successful with your body. This will make it easier for your conscious mind to stay motivated to exercise because the Active Meditation has awakened your conscious mind to take action. When in doubt, close your eyes, take three deep breaths. Play the trailer of the movie with all the amazing new feelings that comes with that new you.

3. *Spiritual Meditation*

What really made a difference in my life was when I started to meditate to go deeper in my spirituality. I truly believe we have all the answers within us. We just need to sit still and listen long enough to hear our inner wisdom. I do a daily meditation for about 20 minutes that includes chakras (energy fields) and ends up at a peaceful and beautiful place where I sit in front of my inner wisdom teacher. Sometimes I just sit passively letting the wisdom flow. Sometimes I bring questions and then I sit actively to listen for answers or words of wisdom. It is quite powerful.

1. Prepare as you did with the Breath & Body Awareness Meditation

2. Place both hands gently on your heart.

3. Bring awareness to the bottom of your spine. Breathe in and out of that location (Root Chakra) as you silently say "I feel grounded. I feel rooted. I feel confident. I feel trust. I feel connected to Mother Earth."

4. Bring awareness to the area around your navel. Breathe in and out of that location (Sacral Chakra) as you silently say "I feel my creativity and my sensuality dance through my body."

5. Bring awareness to the area around your solar plexus (Solar Plexus Chakra). Breathe in and out of that location as you silently say, "I feel my strong willpower propelling me forward to live a fun, healthy, and fulfilling life."

6. Bring awareness to the area around your heart. Breathe in and out of that location (Heart Chakra) as you silently say, "I feel the love, unconditional love and compassion."

7. Bring awareness to the area around your throat. Breathe in and out of that location (Throat Chakra) as you silently say, "I express myself, I speak up, I speak the truth, my voice is authentic."

8. Bring awareness to the area between your eyebrows. Breathe in and out of that location (Third Eye Chakra) as you silently say, "I see the vision, I see my calling, I follow my intuition."

9. Bring awareness to the area around your crown of your head. Breathe in and out of that location (Crown Chakra) as you silently say, "I am connected to a higher power (or use the words that work for you), my inner guide, and my inner wisdom."

10. Inhale and revisit each of the seven chakras, imagining their colors (red, orange, yellow, green, light blue, dark blue, purple) Exhale and imagine a golden white light showering you from head to toes, through all the areas you brought awareness to.

11. Feel how you go deeper and deeper, like an elevator taking you down from the tenth floor to the ground floor. Step out of the elevator into the most beautiful place you can imagine. Use all your five senses to describe it to yourself. Find the most beautiful and inviting spot and make that your meditation spot. Sit down to meditate in your inner world. What do you see in front of you? It can be an object, a person, or just a shape. Imagine that being your wisdom teacher. Ask a question and sit there for the remaining time of your meditation to hear the answer.

12. Finish the meditation the same gentle way as the Breath & Body Awareness Meditation.

Sometimes I decide the question I want to ask ahead of time. When I'm done with the meditation, I write down the answer or any other amazing experiences during this inner journey. Other times the question just appears as I'm meditating. Let it happen. Don't make it happen. That's the magical part of it all.

If you don't have this practice yet, start off the morning with meditation. Why? You will have a better day and be more motivated to stick to an exercise routine. You will have longevity with your life and your exercise plan. Choose one of the three above and stay with the one that resonates with you the most. You will most likely stick to it easier. Repeat it often enough and it will become a wonderful habit you can't live without because you've gotten used to feeling the amazing benefits.

Remember, every thought starts in the mind and can result in a dream of yours coming true. The mind is even more powerful when it works with a healthy body. You now have some tools to make changes in your life. At the end of this book, in Chapter Twelve "Anything is Possible at Any Age," you'll get a chance to dive deeper. It will definitely motivate you to upgrade your life.

Before you move forward to the next chapter, let's take a break to apply some of your inspiration to make changes in life. The actions steps below will be crucial for you to wake up your body and mind throughout your journey of this book.

CHECK-IN #2: AWAKEN YOUR MIND FOR SUCCESS

Stay in the present and imagine what you would like to create in your life right now, both physically and mentally. What one thing can you do from that visualization? What negative voices just popped up in your head? Let's practice changing them into positive affirmations to replace those negatives ones. This list will travel with you throughout the book, keeping the body and mind connection alive. When you do any movements like walking, strength training exercises, and various stretching methods, add these positive affirmations. Pick a few favorite ones and feel the empowering outcome of a strong body and mind. This will get you through anything in life. Get ready. Here you come!

NEGATIVE	POSITIVE
I can't do this.	I can do it.
I'm always lonely.	I'm surrounded by love.
I'm not worth it.	I'm enough.
I'm tired.	I feel light and strong.
I'll walk tomorrow instead.	I'm putting on my sneakers for a 5-minute walk right now – just do it! No more excuses.

My Positive Affirmations

1. _____

2. _____

3. _____

4. _____

5. _____

6. _____

7. _____

8. _____

9. _____

10. _____

Charlene Gorzela - The 6ᵀᴴ DECADE

Being a CEO of a very fast-paced and people-intensive Staffing/Recruiting Firm in Chicago for 26 years, I experienced a feeling of my soul being drained and I knew something had to give. I felt a bit trapped by making an amazing living financially and afraid of the financial insecurity it would bring to my life if I changed careers. Granted, there were many awesome years in my business, but at this time, my soul was telling me it was time to make a major shift.

Suddenly, I was 59 years old and about to expand my company, get larger office space, and sign a ten-year commercial office lease. When I realized I would be close to 70 years old when the lease was over, I started having trouble sleeping. I couldn't stop thinking about the responsibilities I would have... that I did not want. I saw my future and it did not look good. I was full of fear. Something had to shift, or I would be making the biggest mistake in my life... my soul would die, and I would be the shell of me. I knew the jig was up! I asked myself, "If not now, when?" I ended up selling my company. I believe it happened because I let what was going on with the inner me out in the open and that is when the opportunities came. It was like the "Universe" opened up and said a big "Yes" when I woke up to the truth of what was going on within me.

Part of my strategy in life with mind, body, health, and vitality was to work with a fitness expert who trains women and men like me. That is where Malin Svenson comes in. She has helped my life in so many ways. I signed up for her quarterly Holistic Fitness Retreats and use them as a strategy for my health and vitality. I plan on living until I am in my 100's and this means I am only at the half-way point. Now at age 61, my life is very different then it was before. I live in Los Angeles full time. For the first year after I sold the business, I decided to be in a place of allowing and let myself recalibrate to the new me. It took time to untether from my business emotionally, physically, and mentally. I paid attention to me, got quiet, and did not rush into anything. My goal is to live my wildest dreams and how I am doing that today is by doing the next right thing in my life - exploring paths that interest me and that I am pulled to and trust in the mystery of it all. Additionally, I help some non-profits with development and pro-bono work in the recovery field and collaborative housing space for the homeless population.

The best is yet to be and Malin will help take me there... not shuffling but walking tall and proud with a skip in my step!

*~**Charlene Gorzela (age 61), Los Angeles***

"If I had known I was going to live this long,
I would have taken better care of myself."
~**Mae West**

CHAPTER 3:

Put on Your C.A.P. - No More Joint Worry!

Now that your mind has been awakened, let's move into waking up your body. Time to continue the journey of feeding your body and brain good information on how to move correctly to minimize wear and tear on the joints. This will eliminate any fears you may have had about hurting your body while exercising. It's quite simple. All you have to do is to put on the Nordic Body C.A.P. - Core, Alignment, and Posture - and be aware of your body on a daily basis. This is the only body we have or will receive in this lifetime. We want it to last.

"What? I have to move correctly, too? It's not enough to just move? My body has been like this all my life! It's not going to change!" Trust me, I am not suggesting anything dramatic which is the beauty of the Nordic Body C.A.P. Radical change is always unwise. Your body has adjusted itself to be the way it is today. If we were to change anything dramatically, those actions may end up hurting you more than benefitting you. All we are doing is increasing your awareness to prevent any increased tension on already compromised areas of your body.

When you're done with this chapter, you will probably hear my voice saying, "Put on your C.A.P." prior to any movements. The fundamentals behind these three magical letters will increase your body awareness plus promote correct movement. Better yet, it can help improve your movement mechanics to decrease wear and tear on your joints. Sound good? Wonderful. This will be your quick checklist before you pick up your kids, grandkids, nieces, nephews, pets, bags of groceries and when you perform any other daily activities.

C is for CORE

Unless you have lived under a rock for the past 20 years, you have heard the word core. You probably also know it's good to have a strong core to protect, for example, your lower back. I'm not going to explain in depth the core. For now, just think about the core as being the center of your body, including your buttocks and the abdominal area. Let's mainly focus on how to activate the core so you can use it. Everything starts with an active core. Before you lift an arm or a leg, the body is wired to activate the core first before moving a limb. People that are not wired like that may experience more pain, especially in the lower back. Let's get you wired up correctly.

1. Lie face up on the floor with bent knees and both feet firmly on the floor.

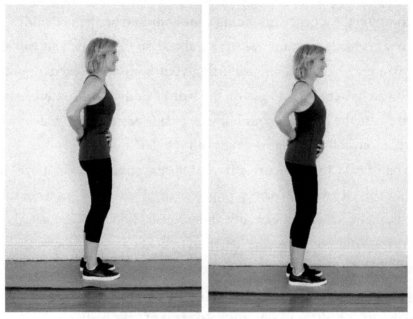

Flatten   *Arch*

2. Gently, like a 10% range of motion, flatten your back. Then gently release and if your lower back allows it, maybe even arch a little bit. Gently! Go back and forth from flattening to releasing/gently arching. If everything feels ok, you can turn it up a notch to 20% and maybe even gradually take it up to a 100% range of motion. This movement is called a **pelvic tilt**. I use it for three reasons

a. To awaken the lower back

b. To check in to make sure the back stays happy after some specific strength training exercises

c. To find the neutral pelvis position

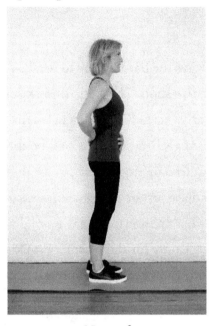

Neutral

3. You are going to use the pelvic tilt now for finding your **neutral pelvis**. Find a happy medium between the flat and arched position of your lower back. When you have found the neutral position, **lock it by gently pulling in the navel**. What happens if you pull in the navel too much? Yes, the back flattens. You don't want that unless you're stretching your front thighs. More about that in Chapter Nine.

By finding your neutral pelvis position and locking it by gently pulling in your navel, you have created a girdle. This is your own internal protection. Have you ever seen bodybuilders, physical labor workers, or people with lower back pain wear a wide serious belt or brace around the waist? That is an external girdle. The purpose is the same - to give support to your lower back area.

I had you lie down to activate your core because it is easier to do pelvic tilts lying down the first time. This is of course not always practical. Practice the same steps standing up or up against a wall. The wall can act as the floor. Move your feet slightly away from the wall and keep your knees slightly bent. Eventually this should become second nature to you - to find your neutral pelvis and to activate the core in any position - sitting, lying, or standing.

A is for Alignment

For some reason, this is always the hardest one to recall. Think about bringing your car in for alignment at the tire shop. The same thing goes for your body. We have to keep it aligned to avoid any excess wear and tear on the joints. It's basically about stacking the joints on top of each other. This will be difficult if you have knock-knees, extremely turned out feet, or any other extreme deviations. Again, we are not here to make dramatic changes; just bringing awareness to your body to ensure the deviations don't get worse. Let's align your body from down and up.

1. Stand in front of a mirror only for the reason of looking at your joints.
2. Keep your feet hip-width apart and preferably barefooted.
3. If it doesn't cause any pain or tension, try to keep all ten toes pointing straight ahead.
4. Standing still, gently roll the **feet** sideways. Tilt them in so they are flat and tilt them out so the arch lifts. Just like a neutral pelvis, find a neutral arch. Not flat and not arched.
5. Move up to your **knees** and observe your kneecaps. Are they looking straight ahead, in or out? The knees are just the slave to the ankle and the hip unless you've had an acute knee injury. Whatever happens in the ankle or hip affects the position of the knee. Try rotating your thighs out and in. Can you feel how that affects the foot arches? Yes, for example if your knees are pointing in, it's very likely that your arches are more on the flatter side. Everything is caving in. Probably the hip(s) as well. See if you can, ever so slightly, rotate those thighs out to gently lift the arches without causing any excess weight on the outside of the foot. It's a gentle correction. Can you feel how suddenly the lazy buttocks woke up and fired up? Yes! In a perfect world we are aiming to have those kneecaps looking straight ahead like headlights of a car.

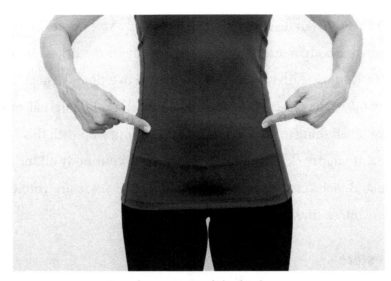

Last bony area of the hipbones

6. Move up to your **hips** and figure out what it means to stand hip-width apart. Place your fingers on top of your right and left hipbones and follow the ridges until you hit the softer abdominal area. That last bony area of the hipbone determines hip-width apart. Take three invisible stickers. Put the first "sticker," which we will call number 1, on that last bony part. Take another "sticker," which we will call number 2, and place that one in the middle of your kneecap. Take the third "sticker," number 3, and place that on your second toe. Do it simultaneously on both legs. The numbers 1-3 should (almost) always line up. Standing hip width apart means that your joints are stacked on top of each other. Hip joint over the knee joint over the ankle joint. Phew! Glad that's done. Being out of alignment is for chiropractors and physical therapists to correct. My alignment awareness exercises are a simple way of making you aware to align your joints to your best ability so you can move your body correctly, efficiently, and pain-free.

7. Wait, there's more! We have the whole **upper body** too. No worries - it's super simple compared to aligning the lower part. The only thing you need to watch for in the mirror is to make sure your shoulders are even and that one is not slanted. If one shoulder is higher or lower than the other one, it usually shows up in your hands being uneven as well. Make sense, right? If your right shoulder is lower, the hand is usually lower as well. You may even lean to the right.

Isn't this fun? To discover parts of your body you never thought mattered? Every bit of your body matters. We sometimes say in the fitness industry that we only have ONE muscle, the fascia. It's the connective tissue beneath the skin that attaches, stabilizes, encloses, and separates muscles and internal organs. Think plastic wrap. Everything in your whole body is wrapped up with this "plastic wrap" called fascia. If your neck gets injured, it can affect your body all the way down to your ankle and vice versa because the neck and the ankle are connected via this fascia. Pretty interesting, right?

P is for Posture

Observing how people walk, stand, and sit can give you information about that person before you even talk to them. Posture is a big part of that indicator. A shy person may round their shoulders, whereas a confident person may open the chest bringing the shoulder blades down and together. Try walking around with those two different postures. How does it make you feel? Shy and timid with rounded shoulders, rounded back, and head down? Secure, confident, and on top of the world when you straightened up and walked around with your head high? Emotions affect us physically, I'm sure you can see and feel that. Next time you feel a little bit down, explore changing your posture to see if you can feel better. Even a smile will make you feel better. According to *Psychology Today*, the feel-good neurotransmitters— dopamine, endorphins, and serotonin—are all released when we smile. This can also lower your heart rate, blood pressure, and relax your body

1. Stand in front of a mirror with an activated core and aligned body.
2. Move the shoulders blades ("wings") up towards your ears and then pull them down away from your ears. Keep them down.
3. Move the shoulders blades forward (rounded back) and then bring them back softly together (open chest). Keep them slightly retracted (slightly together).
4. The palms of your hands should now be facing your thighs. If the front of your hands are facing forward, you need to retract the shoulder blades more.

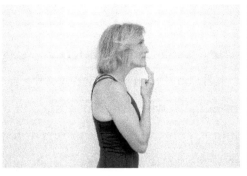
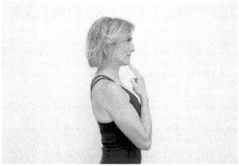

Head forward   *Gently push your head back.*

5. Place two fingers on your chin and gently push your head back. The optimal position is to have the ears lined up with shoulders.

6. Imagine pulling a string up from the crown of your head to elongate your whole spine - from the pelvis all the way up to the neck.

Eventually you only need to think about that imaginary string pulling you up to get into a better posture. This natural traction will help make space for nerves and blood vessels to do their job optimally. You'll be able to assist the natural flow in your body without any interruptions like a pinched nerve, which we all know can be quite painful.

The secret to keeping your C.A.P. on is strength. Yes, it takes **strength** to constantly fight gravity. To stand up straight, to sit up straight, and to move with good posture. We'll cover that in Chapter Seven "Strong is the New Sexy." First let's apply C.A.P when you go for a leisure walk in the next chapter "Every Steps Counts." Enjoy moving your body!

CHECK-IN# 3: PUT ON YOUR C.A.P

C.A.P was created to be a checklist for all my clients to apply before any exercise and/or daily activities. It looks like a lot of work, but if you break it down to practice one at a time, it becomes quite natural. Eventually, when you say or hear "Put on your C.A.P" your body will respond almost automatically by getting into that optimal position to prevent wear and tear of the joints. Sound good? I thought so. Who doesn't want to save their joints? Here we go.

1. C stands for Core - practice activating your core to protect your lower back.

2. A stands for Alignment - practice getting everything lined up evenly in your body to prevent potential injuries.

3. P stands for Posture - practice proper posture to lengthen the spine to give space for nerves, rescuing them from getting pinched.

By just simply putting your C.A.P on, you feel taller, more confident, and empowered. This is your power position. You are ready for anything!

*"A journey of a thousand miles
must begin with a single step."*

~Lao Tzu

CHAPTER 4:

Every Step Counts

Now that you know how to safely move your body, let's move it already! When you hear the word "exercise," do you feel immediate resistance? You're not alone. How do you feel when you hear "movement?" Sounds more fun and less of an effort, right? Great, let's talk about moving your body. There are tons of opportunities throughout the day to move your body for health benefits without having to put on your workout clothes. After this chapter, you will have a whole list of easy options to choose from.

Today we are all about convenience. You can make a living without having to ever leave your home. Everything from books to food can be ordered online. You can do work-related video conferencing with a professional top on, but your bottoms are pajamas. Some of the benefits with this lifestyle can be that we don't have to be stuck in traffic with a car polluting our planet and we get to spend more quality time with our loved ones. However, there are also many disadvantages to never leaving the house - especially in regard to our health. The biggest downside is that we tend to not move our bodies. There's no incentive, unless you were brought up to integrate an active lifestyle to naturally be part of your life, like brushing your teeth. Even if you don't work from home, the "not-moving-your-body" problem is quite widely spread. We sit in our cars, driving to work or running errands. We sit on an office chair at work in front of the computer. When we get home, we sit down on the couch to watch either a TV screen or yet another computer screen for entertainment. The problem with all this sitting is that the body **was made to move**. That's why we have joints - to move. If we don't move the body, it will not operate optimally.

In the late 1890's, pedestrians dominated the roads and cars were rare. If you wanted to get anything done you walked, took a horse carriage, or a streetcar. People moved their bodies without a second thought because it was the way of life. If you go just 100 years back to the roaring 1920's, the lifespan on average was only 54 years compared to 77 years today. The advancement of technology and medicine have us all living longer. The question is, how's your quality of life going to be for those additional years? Will you be bedridden, or will you have freedom of movement? Will you remember what your loved ones look like or will your brain be in a constant fog? Regardless of the unpredictable outcome, it's always best to be your strongest in both body and mind to face any future challenges. Evaluate your body at the age you are. Whether it's in your 50's or your 90's, you can develop ease of body movement and an active healthy lifestyle. No age is too late.

Have you heard that "Sitting is the New Smoking?" On average, Americans **sit** for 11 hours each day. According to the Mayo Clinic, research has linked sitting for long periods of time with a number of health concerns like obesity, increased blood pressure, blood sugar, cholesterol, body fat around the waist, and increased risk of death from cardiovascular disease and cancer. Many studies have shown that if you sit for more than eight hours a day with no physical activity you have a risk of dying similar to the risks of dying caused by obesity and smoking. In summary, less sitting and more moving overall contributes to better health. In fact, right now, let's take a break from reading this book to move. Keep it simple. Stand up and stretch your arms up to the ceiling. How does that feel?

You may experience some stiffness when you stand up after sitting for a long time. This can be caused by the front hip muscles called hip flexors. When you sit, they shorten. In turn, the opposite muscles, the buttocks, they lengthen and weaken. What does this mean? The buttocks "fall asleep" when you sit too long. By the time you're ready to stand up, they are not awake enough to help out, thus it feels strenuous and stiff to stand up. A trick is to tighten and relax your buttocks repeatedly 5-10 times prior to standing. This will awaken them a little bit better. The best solution is to not sit so long but to stand up every 30 minutes. This will naturally stretch the hip flexors and keep the buttocks more alert.

I used to say, "Squeeze your buttocks" with my clients.

"I can't do that! What will people think?" one client responded.

I looked at her strangely. "Nobody will notice that you're tightening and releasing your buttocks while sitting."

Her reaction was pure laughter. Now I was even more confused. Finally, when she was able to speak in between her wonderful giggles, it was clear that she thought I was instructing her to squeeze her buttocks with her hands. I started to laugh too, picturing my poor client at the dinner table squeezing her buttocks with her hands prior to standing.

A sedentary (excessive sitting) lifestyle on planet Earth can have risks equal to being in space and experiencing gravity deprivation. Astronauts in space float around because there's no gravity to fight or resist. Though they are in top shape physically, they lose bone density and muscle strength. When they return to Earth, they have problems walking. The reason is they have been weightless for many months. We can all learn from this - if you don't use it, you lose it. Weightlessness inflicts many bodily systems. Excessive sitting removes the body from its natural condition of constantly resisting gravity. Staying immobile has the same effect as being weightless - it rapidly ages the body and promotes poor health.

A sedentary lifestyle has many detrimental effects on our health:

- Physical inactivity is linked to more than 5 million deaths worldwide per year, more than those caused by smoking.
- Physical inactivity can lead to obesity and Type 2 diabetes.
- 80 percent of adult Americans do not get the recommended amounts of exercise each week.
- Ages 65 and older are least likely to engage in physical activity.

  — *Study from Centers for Disease Control and Prevention (CDC) May 2013*

Do you want to delay the effects of aging? The key to reversing the damage of sedentary living is to put gravity back in your life through frequent, non-strenuous actions that resist the force of gravity throughout the day.

10 Ways to Increase Daily Movement – (choose the one(s) that work for you)

1. Walk and talk with a friend instead of sitting and talking.
2. Include walking when you make dates for dinner, coffee, etc.
3. When you're on the phone, move around.
4. Take the stairs instead of the escalator and elevator.
5. Park your car far away from the entrance to the store.
6. Go for an evening walk before you settle in at home.
7. Set the alarm every hour to stand up to go for a 5-minute walk.
8. Instead of emailing or texting your co-worker a message, walk over to his/her desk.
9. Walk your dog instead of asking someone else to do it.
10. Put on some music you love and move your body.

There are so many health benefits from moving your body. Let's talk about energy. When you sit, you use less energy (calories) than you do when you stand or move. The impact of movement — even leisurely movement — can be profound. For starters, you'll burn more calories. This might lead to weight loss and increased energy (endurance). Also, physical activity helps maintain muscle and bone strength, your ability to move, and your mental well-being, especially as you age.

Do you take moving your body for granted? I want you to stop right now and be grateful for your body. Instead of complaining about taking care of your temple (your body), think about moving your body as a privilege. Yes, that's right, a privilege. If someone who is bound to a wheelchair due to MS was given one minute of freedom, do you think they would keep sitting? I don't think so! They would stand up, walk, jump, dance, run, and be so grateful to be free and able to move their body. It is so easy to complain about things we don't have that we forget to be grateful for the things we do have. If you are fortunate enough to have a body that can move - move it! We reviewed in Chapter One the excuses that may hold you back, and one of them being time. Make time. Prioritize yourself. Start with one of the ten ways to increase your daily movement.

Sometimes what drives us can be quite surprising. Maybe it's money. One person found a cheaper parking structure one mile away from work. Instead of using the expensive parking structure at work, he walked two miles daily - to and from work. He automatically started to lose excess body weight. His goal was not to get in shape. His goal was to save money. His incentive was so strong to save money that he saved his health as well. Now, that's a nice bonus!

What is your incentive? Maybe you have a role model? A grandmother who was active and alert until her last breath? Maybe you want to be like her? Live life with quality and independence. Invest into your health today to reap the benefits tomorrow at an older age. Close your eyes and imagine yourself at age 90. Use the visualization skills in Chapter Two. How do you feel? What does your 90-year-old self tell your younger self today? Listen to that wisdom and apply it. If you can't hear anything, then listen to May West's quote of wisdom: "If I'd known I was going to live this long, I'd have taken better care of myself."

Preparation is key to success. Prepare the evening prior. Prepare when you will move and exercise the next day. If you decide to do some body movement in the morning, decide what you will do, and make sure to set time aside for that. If you decide to exercise in the morning, then put out your workout clothes before going to bed. Make sure you get everything out, so you don't have to run around in the morning to look for the socks. That way, there is no time to change your mind. Ignore the voices saying, "Go back to bed." Instead, don't think - make the NIKE slogan "Just do it!" your mantra.

How we start our morning will affect the rest of our day. How do you start your morning? Is there anything in your morning routine – any habits you would like to change that can help you lead a healthier lifestyle? Can you reduce the stress in the morning? Meditate? Can you delegate tasks to other family members so you can have more time to yourself? Can you add some exercise/movement into your morning routine?

Every Step Counts

A pedometer is an easy way to keep you on track and motivated to move more and to take more steps. At the end of the day, you can have a lot of steps or not that many on your pedometer. The important thing is to start somewhere. Start with a baseline and then build on that - add more steps daily. 10,000 steps are the recommendation for health benefits. Don't freak out if you only have 500 steps. You have to start somewhere. Every journey starts with a first step. If you don't want to keep track of your steps, then keep track of either distance or time. You have to have some kind of measurement. Any time we set goals, they have to be specific and measurable. Since we all take different lengths of steps, it's difficult to say exactly how much certain steps equal in distance. I would say on average 1500-2000 steps is about a mile. And timewise, that's approximately 15-20 minutes.

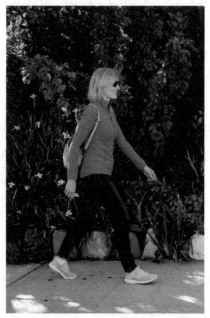

Walk instead of driving your car to everything locally

Growing up in Sweden, I naturally led an active lifestyle. Locally, I used my legs to walk or bike as the main transportation to everything. When I had to go to another city, I used public transportation like the bus or the train. Though I did get my driver's license at age 18, I never owned a car until I moved to Los Angeles at age

28. However, I ended up settling down in my paradise – the city of Santa Monica - because I could easily sustain an active lifestyle just like I did in Sweden.

It was very bizarre to me to see people in Los Angeles drive to a gym (no name to be mentioned…), valet their car, and then go into the gym and walk on the treadmill. Hmm… what's strange about that picture? I realized then that it is not that people can't walk in this city, but it is their mental attitude towards walking. They don't even think about the possibility of walking instead of driving. They were not brought up that way. If you are one of those people, you can make a change. The American car culture has encouraged Americans to drive their cars to everything all the time - even for a block. I sometimes see clients drive to the gym from their homes 200 feet away. You can just imagine my fun conversations with them. Their reasons are that they are on their way to something afterwards or they came back from something. Park your car at home and walk down here. Take advantage of the opportunity to move your body. Every step counts!

Though a lot of American cities do not promote walking and biking safely, I have seen a change for the better since I first arrived in 1989. My mission to help create and promote walking-friendly communities doesn't seem that impossible anymore. (see Adopt-A-Walk in the appendix). The trend today seems to be a return to a carless society, building an infrastructure to where we can walk and bike to everything. Don't look at that trend as if we are going backwards. Instead, we are finally moving forward and becoming smarter in caring both about the health of our bodies and our planet. Living in a city made for pedestrians will make it so much easier to move around. If you have ever been to New York or a city in Europe, you will find yourself walking and moving your body much more than what you may be used to. Those cities were built for pedestrians because they were built before we had cars.

Just like you increased, in Chapter Two, your awareness of the importance of having a mindset aligned with your goals, I cannot stress enough the importance of leading an active lifestyle to reach your health goals. I have given you ways to incorporate more movement into your daily life to more easily achieve your health goals. If you are trying out being healthy for the first time, this is a wonderful way to start.

An active lifestyle means that you move your body physically without having to put on your workout clothes. This is also for you who do work out. If you go to the gym for one hour a day, but then sit on your butt for the rest of the day, it is not healthy. The joints will be cranky, your muscles will feel stiff, and your posture is in danger. The body was made to move - there is no way around it. The instructions are to move it. Move it in a productive way to avoid extra wear and tear. Listen for complaints from your body - if something aches, do something about it. In the next chapter I will show you how to roll your aches away. In the meantime, keep moving.

CHECK-IN# 4: EVERY STEP COUNTS

Check the **10 ways to increase daily movement** list earlier in this chapter. Try out one new way for a week. Add your own ideas on how to increase your steps. Voila, before you know it, you'll be moving your body and feeling so much better. That's what it's all about, right? To feel your best! To feel even better, repeat a positive affirmation (Chapter Two) while moving your body. Feel how you awaken BOTH your body and mind.

My "Ways to Increase Daily Movement" List

1. _____

2. _____

3. _____

4. _____

5. _____

"It always seems impossible

until it's done."

~Nelson Mandela

CHAPTER 5:

Roll Away Your Aches and Pains

Now that you have started to wake up your body a little bit more, you may be surprised by some aches and pains showing up. Not to worry, it is quite normal if you haven't moved your body for awhile. You are at the perfect place to receive solutions on how to literally roll away some of those newly found aches and pains. Maybe you even have some old pains that have created tons of resistance for you to move your body at all up until this point in your life. After this chapter, you will feel much more freedom of movement in your body and I promise you will be totally excited about the fact that a few minutes of rolling a day will make such a huge difference in your life. You will suddenly be able to do activities that you didn't dare to do before due to aches and pains, and you will have a better-quality existence.

How many of you blame aches and pains on age? Yes, it's quite easy to jump to that conclusion. Accusing the aging process is a shortcut that everyone around you accepts. However, this also allows you to assume your achy body will be part of your life without looking into any solutions. That mindset is not empowering. Now, some of the pain can of course be caused by age since our body is a machine that eventually will break down from wear and tear. However, some of the pain can be prevented and even cured. Are you ready to explore? Are you ready to take action towards a new pain-free life?

Nordic Body Reboot Program™

As an ex-massage therapist for ten years and a fitness trainer since 1992, I have developed the Nordic Body Reboot Program™ which consists of three simple steps: **Release, Correct and Load**. I would like to share it with you, so you have a tool to deal with aches and pains.

---

1. **The first step is RELEASE and the purpose is twofold:**
   a. Release tension in a specific muscle using a **trigger release** tool,
   b. Followed by **static stretching** (i.e. holding a stretch for 30 seconds) to get that specific muscle back to its optimal length.

If you have a knot or stiffness in your muscles, most of you would probably do static stretching first on the muscle, right? Now imagine a knot on a rope. What happens if you keep pulling on the rope? Yes, it gets tighter. Instead of doing static stretching first, you want to apply pressure to the knot in your muscles to get a release. I have been doing it on a regular basis since 2000. Back then, I couldn't sleep at night because my right ankle was so painful due to an old athletic injury. After just a couple of weeks of doing trigger release, I was practically pain free.

What trigger release tool should you use? Since 2000, I have tried tons of tools that can help anyone at any time. A soft foam roller is great for beginners. When you get used to that pressure, you can move onto the harder surfaces or even uneven surfaces. There are also vibrational trigger release tools (foam rollers, balls, massage machines) that can go deeper, and they can be used sitting if you can't lie down on the floor.

A trigger release tool can be as simple as a tennis ball. Other specific trigger release balls have been developed. You have the Tiger Ball, which is great to use if you can't lie down on the floor. Put it on the wall and lean on it. There are two bands to hold on to so it doesn't fall off the wall. A tennis ball can be used on the wall as well, but the rubber surface of the Tiger Ball makes it easier to stay steady and not slide around. Finally, you have the massage stick, which can easily be used if you can't lie down on the floor. Though it feels like you're rolling the dough, I wouldn't try using a rolling pin. Let's keep the kitchen tools in the kitchen. Go to https://nordicbody.com/wakeup to watch the video where I present various trigger release tools. As you can see in the video, there are different tools of trigger release - something for everyone. All of you probably have access to a tennis ball – start with that. And enjoy rolling your aches and pains away and know that it works wonders.

There is a famous muscle called piriformis located on your behind. Though it is a small muscle compared to the huge gluteus maximus muscle, it can really cause problems if we don't keep it loose. It runs very close to a nerve – the sciatic nerve. If the piriformis muscle is too tight, it can put pressure on the nerve, and we can be in a lot of pain and feel it all the way down the side of the leg. There is a stretch for the piriformis muscle, and you can do it sitting down in a chair, standing up using poles, or lying down on your back with or without a wall, or lying down on your stomach.

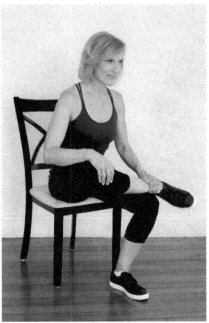 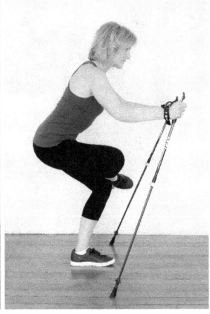

1. Stretching the piriformis muscle sitting on a chair   *2. Stretching the piriformis standing up using poles*

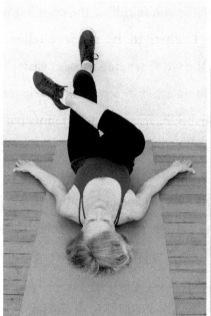 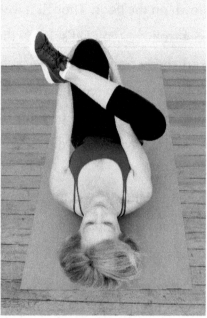

*3. Stretching the piriformis lying
down on your back with a wall*

*4. Stretching the piriformis lying
down on your back without a wall*

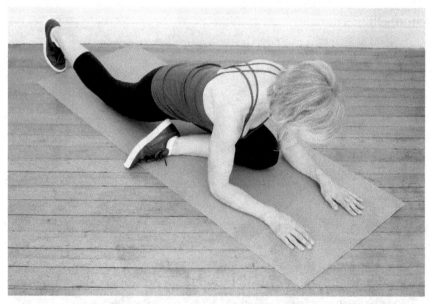

5. Stretching the piriformis lying down on your stomach

Resistance to doing trigger release can be due to a too-painful introduction. That's why it's important to choose the buttocks as the first muscle to explore to prevent you from swearing you will never do that again. Let's do a test by creating a baseline so you can see how effective trigger release really can be to encourage you to continue.

Test Tightness and Trigger Release:

1. Do a piriformis stretch (choose one of the 5 listed above) for 5 seconds on the right leg and then 5 seconds on the left leg. Determine which one is tighter. Use that one as a baseline. If they are equally tight, use both as a baseline.

2. Apply the trigger release technique on either the left or right buttock or both if they are equally tight. If you don't have any trigger release tools, just use your hand, thumb, or knuckles to massage the area that is tight in your buttocks.

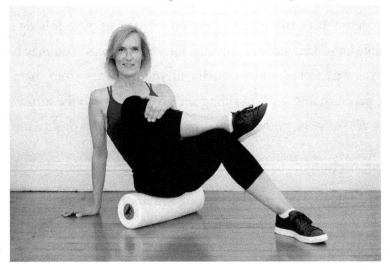

Trigger release technique on right buttock using a foam roller

3. Return to stretch the piriformis on the leg that was tighter to see if you can go any further.

Trigger Release is one of the most important parts of the Nordic Body Reboot Program™, but it can be confusing at first. You may think that your muscles feel fine, but once you foam roll out your right buttock, there is a pain that never appeared to be a problem before. You think, wait, I am here to get fewer aches, not find more. Yet…. this step is about exploring and getting familiar with the muscles in your body to increase your awareness. Through Trigger Release, you get to know your body in a much deeper way. Unfortunately, that means unearthing aches and pains that were previously unattended. Don't make me the bad guy, because I can assure you, in the long run, you will be happy you discovered and worked on these dormant aches. That's why I say trigger release can prevent future injuries. If your hips are currently not hurting on a daily basis, but foam rolling the buttocks muscles hurts, you may actually be doing yourself a great service of continuing doing trigger release on the buttocks to prevent the hips from ever causing you pain. In brief, if you could take care of that sensitivity now, you may prevent it from ever turning into pain when moving your body. I don't expect you to go climb Mount Kilimanjaro, but maybe you want to try dance lessons, swim in the ocean, or lift up your kids without having to stay in bed for three days after. How can we do this as we age? Reboot your body and mind on a regular basis. I'm in! Are you?

Wonderful! Let's take action to explore what areas of your body may be hiding some valuable information about potential future pain areas. You may be very excited, but once you start feeling the sensitivity in your muscles from foam rolling, your excitement may turn into some moaning and groaning due to the surprising sensitivity. No worries. We will start gently. Nothing works well when it is pushed too hard, too fast.

Release Instructions:

As I mentioned above, I recommend starting with the buttock muscles. If you start with the IT band (on the outside side of each leg) I promise you will stop doing trigger release because it will be too painful and too shocking. Wherever you start on the body, use these 2 steps, and then repeat.

1. **Explore** your muscles to find sensitive spots by rolling around on the muscle using the trigger release tool of your choice. Keep the muscle you're doing trigger release on as relaxed as possible. When you've found a spot, **hang out** there and apply some pressure for 20-60 seconds. Make sure you can breathe. If it's too painful, lighten up the pressure or move to the next spot. If it radiates, move the trigger release tool a few millimeters away to avoid putting pressure on the nerves. You're not looking for a 100% release, but maybe 50-70%. When you feel that **release,** move to the next sensitive place and repeat.

2. Now that the knots of that muscle have been released as much as possible, continue to release the muscle by doing static stretching to **lengthen** the muscle to its normal length or beyond if necessary. Hold for 30 seconds. Eventually you will learn which ones are tight and which side (right or left) is tighter and you can focus on static stretching on those specific muscles and sides.

Look at the photos below to find out where to do **trigger release** on certain muscles **followed by static stretching**.

TRIGGER RELEASE	**STATIC STRETCH**

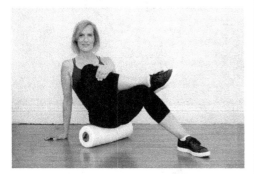

Trigger Release the buttock

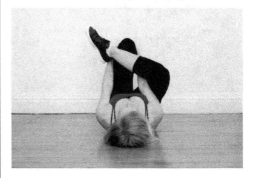

Static Stretch the piriformis

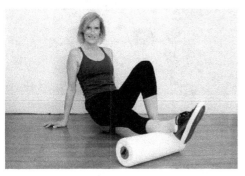

Trigger Release the calf…

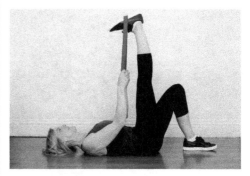

Static Stretch the calf and the hamstring

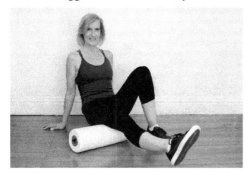

…. and the hamstring

TRIGGER RELEASE	**STATIC STRETCH**

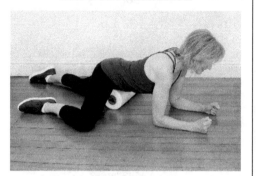

Trigger Release the quadriceps

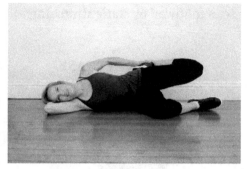

Static Stretch the quadriceps (front thigh)

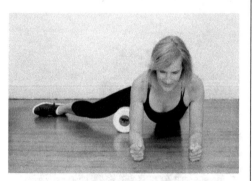

Trigger Release the inner thigh

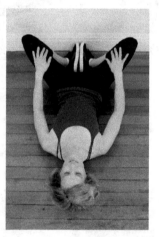

Static Stretch the inner thighs

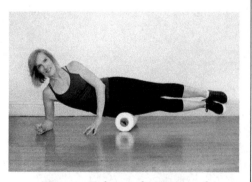

Trigger Release the IT Band

(side of the leg)

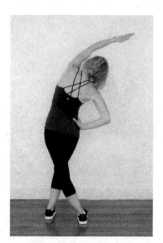

Static Stretch the IT Band

WAKE UP Your Body + Mind After 50

---

2. The second step is CORRECT, and the purpose is to:
Reprogram your muscles by awakening the communication between the nerves and the muscles using corrective exercises.

When the knot gets released from trigger release, the blood circulation increases. Now fresh blood can enter, and the waste products can be removed. Voila, you have more functioning muscle fibers. But though they are free from being tangled up in a knot, they are also lost and confused. They've been asleep for so long that they have forgotten their job description. Now that they are awake, you need to reprogram and retrain them by basically teaching them how to fire (how to work).

If you skip this step, your muscles will most likely go back to the old way and that knot will most likely start building up again. After you have done trigger release + static stretching on as many muscles as possible, it is time to do the corrective exercises.

First, do a corrective exercise called **bridge**, followed by a corrective exercise called **plank**. Both should be done isometrically, which means you just hold the position. There's no movement. The important thing is to get into the correct position to provide correct information to the muscles and nerves. In addition to being corrective exercises they are both great core strength exercises. You get two benefits for one effort. A way to strengthen your abs and butt without really committing. Pretty sneaky!

Hold the position for 30-60 seconds to give the muscle fibers a chance to realign and to start functioning fully again. Having worked with the 50+ population since 1992, I have seen clients able and not able to lift their buttocks off the floor, bench, or bed. Every client who has struggled with lifting their hips up is struggling with their walk. They can't walk more than a few minutes, or they have to use a cane, a walker, or maybe even a wheelchair because they can't walk at all. Please, always aim to be able to do a bridge at any stage of your life.

Correct Instructions:

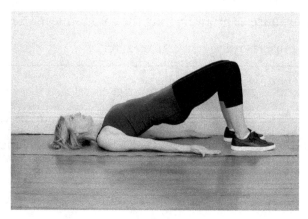

Bridge

How to do a **bridge** correctly:

1. Lie on the floor, on a bench, or in bed.

2. Keep your feet hip-width apart. Line up hip, knee, and 2nd toe.

3. Do a few *gentle* pelvic tilts to make sure your lower back is happy and to find your neutral spine. Find a happy medium between the flat and arched back. Lock the neutral position by lightly pulling in the navel. Now you have created your own girdle.

4. Gentle squeeze your buttocks and make sure nothing hurts.

5. Push the heels gently down into the floor, bench, or bed.

6. Continue lifting the hips up as you exhale and lower them as you inhale. Do 5 slow, controlled movements up and down. Explore first with a tiny lift and proceed to a higher lift if it feels good.

7. Make sure the hips are even and stable. They should not be sinking down on one side.

8. Hold the hips at the highest level for 30-60 seconds.

9. If you feel the hamstrings cramping, try to dig the heels deeper into the ground to access the buttocks better.

10. If the cramping does not stop, then stop the exercise. You are gradually building your strength. Eventually you will be able to stay here for 60 seconds. Maybe even by tomorrow, you will be able to hold it longer.

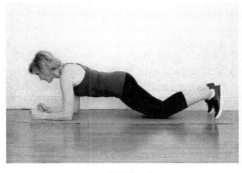 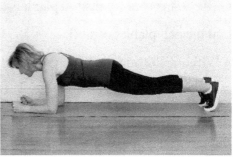

Half Plank   *Full Plank*

How to do a **half plank** and a **full plank** correctly:

1. Start on all fours and come down to your lower arms.

2. Line up your elbows with your shoulder joints. They should be stacked on top of each other.

3. Line up your knees with your hips in a half plank position. They should be stacked on top of each other.

4. Your back should be flat like a table. You should be able to put a plate on your back without it falling off.

5. Do a few _gentle_ pelvic tilts to make sure your lower back is happy and to find your neutral spine. Find a happy medium between the flat and arched back. Lock the neutral position by lightly pulling in the navel. Now you have created your own girdle.

6. Make sure your head is not dropping but lifted so you're looking straight down on the floor. Tuck in your chin and gently push the chin up to get into the proper position.

7. Check in with your shoulder blades. Make sure they are pulled away from your ears and slightly retracted.

8. Imagine something pulling you forward from the crown of your head at the same time something is pulling you backward from the tailbone. There is a nice traction throughout the spine.

9. This position is a half plank and it may be enough for you. When you can stay here for 60 seconds, upgrade to a full plank.

10. The best way to try the full plank is to start with tucking in your toes when you're in the half plank position.

11. Without shifting the hips, gently lift one knee off the floor (keeping the toes on the floor) and stay here for a few seconds. Then bring the knee back down. Repeat the same thing on the other knee. If there are any red flags, meaning if you experience any lower back pain, return to the half plank. Alternating knees can be a great way to slowly build up your core strength to a full plank.

12. When you feel the alternating knee lifts are a piece of cake after 60 seconds, then you are ready to try the full plank.

13. Instead of alternating lifting the knees, you let both knees be off the floor. The second you feel pain anywhere, you return slowly into a half plank for the rest of the time. Maybe the first time you were able to do 10 seconds in a full plank and 50 seconds in a half plank. Next time try to increase the full plank time and decrease the half plank time until one day when you can do a full plank for 60 seconds.

> ### 3. The third step is LOAD and the purpose is twofold:
>
> a. Challenge and fatigue the muscle to get stronger without hurting yourself.
>
> b. Bring awareness to which side is weaker and which is stronger to correct muscular imbalances.

Sometimes we go straight to loading, ignoring aches and pains. You're really doing yourself a disservice. Take one minute to **release** and take one minute to **correct** before you load the muscles and joints. It's that simple. I know people that are workout fanatics, sometimes doing two or more workouts a day long term. They abuse their bodies and limp around with aches and pains. If they just took five minutes a day to do trigger release + static stretching and corrective exercises prior to loading their muscles, they would be in a lot less pain. So, if this is you, wake up - stop the abuse and start honoring and respecting your body. There is a reason our bodies are equipped with pain receptors - they are there to tell us when we are pushing the body too much and too hard. Start listening, really listening, to your body's warning signals! Otherwise, you may end up spending unnecessary money and time on CT scans, X-rays, and MRI's AND you may have made the injury worse by postponing taking care of the pain. Now the healing process will take even longer.

Time to load the muscles individually and see what they're made of. We are going to do single leg bridges and side planks on both the right side and the left side to see if they are equally strong. If you have a weaker side, do two sets on that side. For example, if my right side is weaker than my left side, I start with the right, continue with the left, and then return to do a second set on the right.

I had a 90-year-old client, Ephraim, who improved over the years with single leg bridges. He could do 30 seconds and sometimes more. And at age 90, he was still able to get down and up from the floor. Sounds easy to some of us, but ask anyone who is close to 90 years old if they can get up and down from the floor. I promise you, not a lot of them can do it.

Load Instructions:

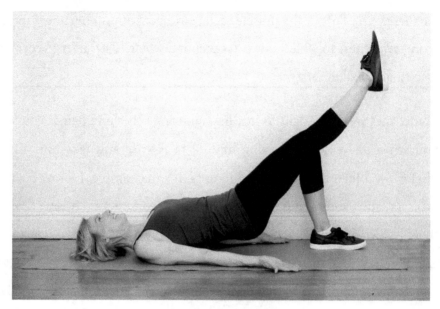

Single Leg Bridge

How to do a **single leg bridge** correctly:

1. Get into the corrective bridge exercise position - feet hip width apart, neutral spine, squeeze the buttocks, push through the heels, and gently lift up the hips high as you exhale.

2. Hold the hips at the top making sure the hips are even and stable. They are not sinking down on one side.

3. Check in with your arms. Keep the arms on the floor to help you stabilize the position. Try keeping the palms facing up and feel how the shoulder blades are away from your ears and down towards your buttocks.

4. Slowly stretch out one leg so the knees of both legs remain at the same height, but the foot of the stretched leg is in the air.

5. This will feel much harder now that only one buttock muscle is making it possible for both hips to stay off the floor. The leg that has the foot on the ground is the working leg.

6. Hold this single leg bridge position for 30-60 seconds.

7. If you feel the hamstrings cramping on the working leg, try to dig the heel deeper into the ground to access the buttock better.

8. If the cramping does not stop, then stop the exercise. You are gradually building your strength. Eventually you will be able to stay here for 60 seconds. Maybe even by tomorrow, you will be able to hold it longer.

9. When you have finished one leg, return both hips to the ground and rest. When you are ready, repeat steps 1-6 on the other leg.

10. Be aware of which one is weaker. Make sure you do 2 sets on the weaker side.

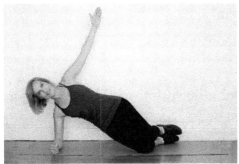 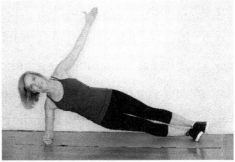

Half Side Plank   *Full Side Plank*

How to do a **half side plank** and a **full side plank** correctly:

1. Lie on either side. Prop yourself up on your arm. Line up shoulder with elbow so the joints are stacked on top of each other. Then line up the elbow with the wrist.

2. Line up both hips so they are stacked on top of each other. The same with the knees and feet.

3. Let's start with a half side plank, which means your knees are bent.

4. Make a fist with your hand and push it slightly into the floor. Make sure you feel like a turtle, elongating your neck and keeping the shoulders away from your ears, and shoulder blades retracted.

5. Bring up the arm that is not on the floor - bring it towards the ceiling keeping the palm facing forward. A common mistake is to fall forward. Keeping the

chest open with the help of that arm plus squeezing your shoulder blades will prevent that falling forward.

6. Now that you're in a perfect position, pull in the navel to activate the core. Exhale and lift your hips up. Only the lower arm, knees, and feet are touching the ground.

7. Imagine something pulling you from the crown of your head at the same time something is pulling you from the tailbone. Through this elongation there is a nice traction throughout the spine.

8. Hold this half side plank position for 30-60 seconds. When you can stay here for 60 seconds, upgrade to a full side plank.

9. To get into the full side plank, straighten your legs so that only the lower arm and your feet are touching the ground.

10. The second you feel pain anywhere, return slowly into a half side plank for the rest of the time. Maybe the first time you were able to do ten seconds in a full side plank and 50 seconds in a half plank. Next time, try to increase the full plank time and decrease the half plank time until one day when you can do a full plank for 60 seconds.

11. When you have finished one side, repeat everything on the other side.

12. Be aware of which side is weaker. Make sure you do 2 sets on the weaker side.

Be patient and know that you can see results at any age. A client of mine, Marilyn, was 80 years young when she came to me with pain in her left hip. The pain was so severe that she could not walk upstairs. After only two weeks of applying to the Nordic Body Reboot Program, she could walk upstairs again pain-free. Now, keep in mind, she was very disciplined and practiced the three steps every day by herself. If you don't do the work, you won't feel the benefits.

Now that you have dealt with some potential pain that may have prevented you from more fun and liberating movements, let's step it up a notch to "Move Dynamically Without Fear" in the next chapter. Enjoy!

CHECK-IN #5: ROLL AWAY YOUR ACHES AND PAINS

Try at least the buttocks muscles. You have nothing to lose but pain and that should be a huge incentive in itself. If you have problems coming down to the floor, use a tennis ball or a Tiger Ball (rubber) up against the wall. It is just as efficient. Same thing with the bridge - you can do that on the bed or on a sturdy couch.

1. Trigger release on the buttocks.

2. Piriformis Static Stretching for the buttocks.

3. Corrective exercising with the bridge, holding it for up to 60 seconds.

4. Loading exercise with a single bridge, holding it for up to 60 seconds.

Now doesn't that feel good to awaken those muscles that may have been asleep for a long time? Why don't you try another part of your body and wake that up as well? Try the calves. You'll be surprised what they have been hiding from you for years.

Delphine Man - The 8TH DECADE

As we age, there will definitely be challenges in many areas of our lives. It is how we handle those challenges that will make a difference if we are still fortunate enough to have a sound mind. I almost gave in to horrible back pain - meaning I stopped moving for four years. That was probably the worst thing I could have done, but I was in so much pain that I didn't know what else to do. Unfortunately, what you don't use, you lose. It was very depressing to see and feel how I became less active and gradually started to lose my muscle strength. It was a vicious cycle. Movement caused pain, but no movement caused decreased strength. Talk about a catch 22!

All my life, I have been very active and adventurous. I grew up in the UK but moved to Los Angeles in 1975, along with my then-husband, who was a very successful screenwriter, and our two children, ages five and seven. Fast forward almost 40 years, when at age 84, I had a horrendous experience when my back went out. It seemed it happened for no reason, but I'm sure it had been building up gradually and this was the straw that broke the camel's back, so to speak. Several friends introduced me to their favorite chiropractor - all without any success. In fact, it got worse and I could hardly move, and I couldn't drive. Anyone living or visiting Los Angeles knows how limiting it is to not be able to drive a car in this town. Then I tried two epidurals (a medical procedure to take away nerve pain) but neither worked. The next seemingly logical step was surgery, which was recommended by a couple of doctors, but fortunately not by my doctor, who, in fact, had a totally different opinion and even begged me not to have surgery. Guess whose advice I followed? Yes, my doctor's - I didn't have surgery.

Eventually my back started to get better and stronger. For 14 years I had done Pilates, but I couldn't do that anymore. I struggled for a year or more and then my friend asked me to join her and work with Malin. What an amazing difference that has made - I now have very little, infrequent back pain. After just 6 weeks of working with Malin, I was able to walk for exercise. Now I walk every morning for about a mile to get my coffee. Malin has been amazing and I am grateful for being able to lead a perfectly normal life. So please, if you have any pain, do not give up and if you can, work with Malin - can't recommend her enough!

~Delphine Mann, age 88, Los Angeles, CA

"We don't stop playing because we grow old.
We grow old because we stop playing."
~George Bernard Shaw

CHAPTER 6:

Move Dynamically Without Fear

You've done trigger release to roll away your aches and pain and, in that process, you also started to reboot your body to have muscles and nerves communicate better. The key is to keep feeding your body with that correct communication and information by always putting on the C.A.P. Now you're ready to step it up to advance your body to be ready for anything, like the Nordic Body Dynamic Drills. Created to be used as part of the warmup prior to a workout, the drills will take you back to your childhood days of hopscotch and other fun games.

Let's explore some more fun and different ways to move your body to keep waking it up. Dig deep into your childhood. What were some of your more delightful memories from the playground or playing with your friends? Go back to that kid within you and reminisce about the movements you were able to do without thinking and without fear. Swinging super high and jump? Sliding down the slide in full speed? Climbing trees?

What happened with that playful kid? When did you stop playing? When did you stop exploring how the body moves? I understand who you are now may not lend itself to playground-type play, but it is the energy of fun and joy that we can bring to the way you move and take walks. I will help you integrate into that exploration more security in your walk and when you move in general.

Coming from an athletic background, I know the value of moving the body in different ways and with different speeds. As a matter of fact, I work out every client of mine as an "athlete" just because to be an athlete you have to be good at almost everything physically. They are very well trained all around. During the workouts with my clients, we cover all aspects of physical training including strength, balance, coordination, speed, flexibility, and reaction to keep the body agile. As we age, we have to stay on top of all aspects of physical training - just like an athlete.

Did you know your body is three-dimensional? That means you can move your body in three directions - straight forward/back, sideways, and rotational. Most of us only move straight forward. The body will get used to this direction only. When and if an unfortunate accident happens, it's most likely to happen in the rotational plane because the body is not used to moving in that direction. Accidents can occur in other planes too, especially when changing surfaces. For example, have you ever walked forward and caught your foot on the carpet when changing from the floor to the carpet? Hopefully, you were able to catch yourself to prevent falling. My clients tell me about incidents of them almost falling, like tripping. Though I may react with upping the "dynamic drills" (body awareness, balance, coordination, speed, reaction) of our training, I also feel relieved about the fact that they were able to prevent the fall.

Just the other day, a client came into her private session with me and said, "Thank you, Malin, for making me do these Dynamic Drills! I almost had a horrible fall the other day coming down the stairs wearing slippery, leather-soled shoes. Miraculously, I managed to regain my balance and I *know* it is due to our training." We looked at each other and took a deep breath of relief and gratitude.

Yes, we can all get lazy about picking up our feet but if something throws us off, it's the ability to react quickly that will save you from falling. Fear of falling is a big concern as people age. You may have heard that a fall can cause death. That doesn't mean that you'll die from the fall itself, but if your bones are not strong enough, you may break (fracture) a hip and some people do not recover from that. Some bones may be so fragile that you can't operate on them. You may have to lie in bed for months to heal. It's a painful and vicious cycle.

As we have established earlier, a sedentary lifestyle decreases bone density and muscle strength. Being bedridden definitely qualifies for a sedentary lifestyle. You are not thinking about the repercussions of falling now and won't until after it happens. That's why I bring these warnings up now, so you have the luxury of doing something about it right this second, before it's too late. As you age, you need **body awareness**, **balance** (physical equilibrium), **coordination, speed,** and **fast reactions** in addition to **strength** (covered in Chapter Seven) and **flexibility** (covered in Chapter Nine) to prevent falls. All in all, your body needs to be agile to prevent falls. Doing the Nordic Body Dynamic Drills, strength training, and stretching on a regular basis will give you these abilities. A lot of the Dynamic Drills in this chapter are about being able to quickly move your feet, pick the feet up from the floor, and have good balance while doing it.

When I work out a client, I move them in all three dimensions to prepare the body for the real world outside the gym. The second you step into a workout session, your body awareness is heightened. You may not consciously keep that increased state of mind after a workout session, but the idea of practicing moving in different directions with different speeds is that your body will be more prone to automatically remember how to react. This way, your body will assist you in getting out of an unpredictable and dangerous situation.

Practicing Nordic Body type Dynamic Drills is something any athlete at any age can do. Applying these moves is not something we should just start doing when we feel our balance is off. We haven't maintained those skills since our playground days. That's why you need to get reacquainted with these movements today to be in tip top shape for tomorrow to assist aging successfully. Included in the Dynamic Drills are movements that challenge, in a fun, way your body awareness, balance, coordination, speed, and reaction.

A Taste of Dynamic Drills

Do these Dynamic Drills to your capacity. Have fun with it and get back to that "playground" without fear of falling. Sometimes it will feel like dancing, which in itself is a great combination of many ingredients in Dynamic Drills. All these new movements have another common denominator - they are great for your brain. One more brain and mind benefit is to integrate some positive affirmations while executing these drills.

Here are a few to get you started:

- "I'm fast!"
- "I am coordinated!"
- "I have fast reactions!"
- "I can do this!"
- "My body is awake and alive!"
- "It is fun playing!"
- "I have energy like a kid!"
- Make up your own that resonate with you.

Add them to the list at the end of Chapter Two so you can easily access them. Hopefully, you already have a few powerful ones you can pull from that Positive Affirmation list.

Pick just one Dynamic Drill and repeat it 1-2 times every week for a month. Then try a different drill.

BODY AWARENESS

How well do you know your body? Knowing your limits, as well as freedom of movement, is crucial as we are aging. Don't wake up one day surprised at not being able to stand up easily from a low couch. Get to know your body from toe to head by doing this Body Awareness Drill. Use some of the movements as a warmup before a workout to prepare your body for moving with more range of motion and with more resistance. Really pay attention to what is easy and what is more difficult. Working on weaknesses is not as fun as working on strengths. However, we are aiming to correct muscular imbalances in your body to have a functioning, pain free, and strong body. Your weaknesses need to be addressed for that freedom of movement to happen as you are aging. Listen to your body.

Let's start by sitting on the edge of a chair with feet flat on the floor. Even if the following ten sitting-down movements may be easy, they build a great base.

Review them at least once until you go straight to the standing up ones. Some of the sitting down and the standing up movements are similar, and they build on each other. Whether you are sitting or standing keep the C.A.P on (Chapter Three).

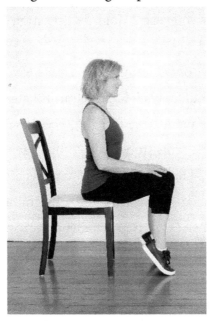

1. Sit on the edge of a chair with feet flat on the floor. Exhale and slowly lift the heels up as high as possible. Aim to come up as high as on your balls of your feet. Stay there two counts and slowly return. Repeat 10 times.

2. Slide out both feet about a foot. Exhale and lift all ten toes towards you so you are only on the heels. Hold that position for 2 counts then slowly return. Repeat 10 times.

3. Slide both feet back to where they are flat on the floor. Straighten one leg and place the center of the heel on the floor. Pull the five toes up towards you and feel a slight stretch on the back of the lower leg. Place both hands on the opposite leg. Lean forward with a straight back. Feel the stretch behind the knee and/or behind the thigh (hamstrings). Hold that position for 2 counts, then slowly return. Repeat 10 times alternating legs (5 on each side).

4. Activate the core by pulling in the navel. Exhale and slowly lift one knee up. Hold that position for 2 counts then slowly return. Repeat 10 times, alternating legs (5 on each side).

5. Circle your shoulders gently and slowly in an up, back, down, and forward motion making the circles as big as possible. Repeat 5-10 times.

6. Clasp both hands. Exhale and lift both arms up toward your head. Aim to have the arms line up with your ears. Hold that position for 2 counts then slowly return. Repeat 10 times.

7. Scoot back in the chair so you feel the upper back touch the back support of the chair. Squeeze your shoulder blades. Let the arms hang on each side of the chair. Turn the hands so the palms face forward. Feel how it's easier to squeeze the shoulder blades. Lift the arms straight up to the side with thumbs pointing up. Stop at shoulder height. This is the start position. Keeping the arms straight, bring the arms together in front of you at shoulder height until the hands touch with palms facing each other. This is the end position. Feel the shoulder blades separate in the back. Return the arms to the starting position and feel the shoulder blades squeeze together. Hold that position for 2 counts. Repeat 5 times.

8. Go back to the same starting position as the previous movement. Keep the shoulder blades in touch with the back support of the chair. Make sure the shoulders are away from the ears and lengthen the neck. Keep this focus as you slowly rotate your head to the right. Hold it for 2 counts then rotate to the left side. Hold it for 2 counts. Return to looking straight ahead. Now tilt the neck - ear to shoulder. Hold it for 2 counts, return, and tilt the neck to the other side. Hold it for 2 counts. Repeat the rotation and tilting of the neck for a total 8-12 times.

9. For the final sitting exercises, we will focus on your wrists and elbows. Bend your elbows, bring your hands together in front of your body, palms facing each other. Lightly push the hands together, straightening the fingers as much as you can. Keeping the shoulders away from your ears, try lifting the elbows up without letting the palms of the hands separate. You should feel a stretch on the inside of the lower arms. Hold it for 2 counts. Release. Repeat 5 times.

10. Let's do the opposite of the previous movement. Turn the hands upside down with the fingers pointing down. Keep the back of the hands touching. Without separating the wrists, try pushing the elbows down. You should feel a stretch on

the front of the lower arms. Hold it for 2 counts. Release. Repeat 5 times. How's your flexibility or stiffness in your elbows and wrists?

Let's continue the Body Awareness Drills, this time standing up. We transition from sitting to standing by learning a simple, yet crucial, technique on how to stand and sit correctly. Apply this awareness every time you get up and down from a chair and you will never have problems getting up or down as you are aging. Sound too simple? Not when you are 90 years old and that is what we have been training for, right?

1. Sit on the edge of a chair with feet flat on the floor. Place your hands on your thighs. Lean forward. Squeeze the buttocks and push heels down into the floor. Keep leaning forward until the butt comes off the chair. Use your legs to stand up and then straighten your back. When you are your tallest, pretend there is a string you can pull up from the crown of your head to get you even taller. Stay here two counts. Reverse and sit down on five counts keeping the weight on the heels and the buttocks. Make sure both knees stay straight ahead like headlights. Repeat standing and sitting 10 times. Think about unfolding and folding your body in a smooth transition.

2. Stand tall with feet hip-width apart. Raise one heel off the floor. Come up as high as you can pain-free. Aim to be on the ball of the foot and maybe even the toes. Hold that position for 2 counts. Repeat a total of 10 times (5 on each side). Exaggerate the range of motion to become familiar with the flexibility or stiffness of your ankles.

3. Now raise both heels at the same time. The slower the better. Pause at the top. Control it down. When you feel confident, add the arms. Bend the elbows, keeping both hands just in front of the shoulders. From that position, straighten the arms up over your head each time the heels come off the floor. Hold the end position for 2 counts. Repeat a total of 10 times. Check in to see how flexible or stiff your shoulder joints are. How is your balance?

4. Gently bend one knee like kicking your butt with your heel. If the quads are tight, you may feel a stretch. Alternate legs. Keep the core active to prevent the lower back from hurting. Before you add the arm movement, make sure the palms face

forward and the fingertips reach down towards the floor. Bring awareness to how this allows the shoulders to move away from the ears. Add lengthening of the neck and you have created a nice natural traction in your neck and shoulder area. Squeeze the shoulder blades. That is the arm position when a knee bends. Move the arms slightly forward, slightly separating the shoulder blades. That is the arm position when a foot lands on the floor. Coordinate arms and legs. It is good for your body and brain. Do a total of 10 (5 on each side). Check the flexibility

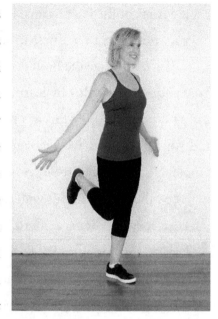

or stiffness of your knee joints and chest. If you want to be really productive, add a neck turn each time you squeeze the shoulder blades together. Alternate sides and alternate with neck tilts. Now you can also check the flexibility or stiffness of your neck.

5. Stand with your feet hip-width apart. Clasp both hands. Activate the core. Lift them over your head. Leave them there. Aim to have the arms by your ears but don't force it if it hurts. Now do a knee lift and lower the clasped hands to touch the knee. Hold it for 2 counts. Return arms up and return the foot down. Repeat 10 times, alternating legs (5 on each side). Check the flexibility or stiffness of your hip and shoulder joints and balance.

6. Focus on only moving the arms. Cross the arms in front of you. Lift the arms up towards the ceiling. At the top, uncross the arms and return them back down on the side of the body. Repeat. Do a total of 10.

7. *Be very careful with this last one if you have any lower back problems or dizziness.* Stand with your feet hip-width apart. Sit down slowly to a squat position (no chair). Continue to lean forward until your fingertips are as close to the floor as possible. Keep all the weight on the legs. There should be no strain in your lower back. Hold this position for 2 counts. Before you return, pull in the navel and curl up one

vertebrae at a time, with the head last, until you are back to standing nice and tall again. Take a break. When you feel ready, repeat it 4 more times.

You have just scanned pretty much all of your joints from ankle to neck. How did that feel? Any surprises of extra tightness somewhere? We have a tendency to forget our joints that are furthest away from the center of the body - ankles, wrists and neck. Now you have checked in with them, keep them flexible and happy. The *Body Awareness* Dynamic Drill is available on video at https://nordicbody.com/wakeup.

BALANCE

Did you know while walking you are practicing balance? There is a brief moment when you are on one leg only. Right before one foot lands, the opposite leg holds up all of you. That's why it's more difficult to walk slower than faster. If I ask you to walk with high knees, you may think that's simple. Do it again and now linger on one leg for 5 seconds. That's harder. That's why having and working on good balance is so important throughout life. When people feel insecure while walking, what do they do? Sometimes they widen the stance and return to how we started to walk as a toddler. Sometimes they add a cane or even a walker. If you have a balance disorder, the information in this section will not always apply to you. We will be dealing with regular imbalances and try to improve them.

Your vision, your hearing, and your ability to know where your body is in space (proprioception) affects your balance. Have you ever seen elderly people looking down at their feet as they walk? Yes, they constantly need to "see" where their feet are in space. My verbal cue to clients that do that is, "Talk to your feet without having to look down to see your feet." Poor proprioception, poor vision, and poor hearing makes it more difficult to keep your balance. Working on the Dynamic Drills below will improve your proprioception. The first one is the easiest and the last one, number ten, is the most difficult one. Honor your body and stay with the one that you can control with a slight challenge. Gradually build it up. If you're challenging yourself too much and you're swaying all over the place, you're doing yourself a disservice. Plus, more importantly, you are jeopardizing your safety. Please be patient and smart. *You can't hurry love or balance.*

One trick to better keep the balance is to think about the leg you're standing on as a solid pillar. The foot of the standing leg is pushing down to Mother Earth while an invisible string from the crown of your head is pulling you up towards Father Sky. It's like two forces pulling you apart in two different directions, making that leg a super solid pillar. All muscles of the standing leg are active and assisting: the calf, the quad (front thigh), the buttock, and the core while keeping a good posture. Some people hyperextend the knee. Avoid that by ever so slightly softening the knee while trying to tighten the quad muscle. If you can get a sense of pulling the kneecap up towards your head, that will further prevent you from hyperextending the knee joint.

Hold each of the positions below for 3-10 seconds before you move onto the next one.

1. Balance on one leg with support.
2. Lunge position (one leg is positioned forward with knee bent and foot flat on the ground while the other leg is positioned behind) with both heels on the floor.

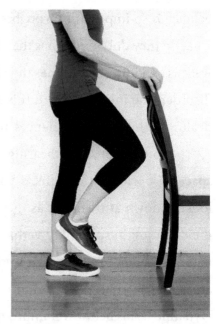

3. Lunge position with heel up on back leg.
4. Balance on one leg without support.
5. Step up onto a step with support.
6. Step up onto a step without support.
7. Step up onto a step and lift opposite leg (knee lift).
8. Step up onto a step and abduct opposite leg (lift sideways).
9. Step up onto a step and rotate opposite leg (knee lift + rotate out)
10. Add an object to stand on that will enhance the instability like a Pillow, Soft Pad, Bosu, or Wobble board. Then repeat 1-9.

SPEED

Having worked with the 50+ population since 1992, I have noticed that some people have only one gear. Think about your car. What if you could drive only in first gear? If you're not familiar with stick shift, that is on average a speed of 5mph (8km per hour). That's nice and slow, but it probably would drive you crazy to drive that slowly for a long time. On the other hand, if you had to get out of a dangerous situation, you could easily stop by pushing on the brakes without generating too much whiplash damage. Nonetheless, what if you had to move fast because somebody was coming towards you at high speed? Yes, you'd shift quickly to 5th gear to get the heck out of there. Same applies to your body machine - let's test drive it to see how fast you can move. Safety first, though. When you're with a trainer, you can probably challenge yourself more. Without a trainer who is not watching every move you make, you want to be more careful.

First, scope out a safe area like a hallway. Make sure there are no obstacles in your way. The ideal length would be around 25 feet (8meters), but shorter distance works as well.

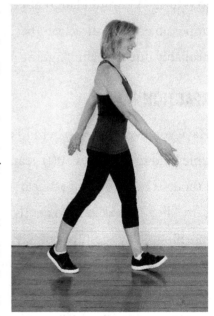

1. Walk straight forward about 25 feet at slow speed. Look straight ahead. If you need to look down, use your eyes instead of bending your neck.

2. Return, walking straight backward about 25 feet at slow speed. If you do not feel safe even at a slow pace, hold onto a wall for support (if you walk down a hallway).

3. Turn to your left, facing a wall (if you walk down a hallway) Walk to the right, taking short side-to-side steps, leading with the right foot. Keep all 10 toes pointing straight ahead. Walking sideways can be tricky for a lot of people. Pick up those feet to avoid any tripping. Walk sideways about 25 feet at slow speed.

4. Return, walking to the left, taking short side-to-side steps, leading with the left foot.

5. Stand in the middle between the two walls. Look straight ahead and choose a specific spot to be your return landmark. Slowly rotate, in a small circle, to your right, taking short rotational steps leading with the right foot.

6. As you return to your "landmark," change directions. Slowly rotate to your left until you reach the landmark again.

7. Repeat 1-6 at a moderate speed

8. Repeat 1-6 at a fast, but safe, speed.

The faster you go in rotation, the dizzier you'll get. Do it safely. Avoid bending your neck to look down. That will only make you even more dizzy. I remember back in Sweden when we did games during the summertime celebrating Midsummer (the longest day of the year). One game was to run forward to a short pole in the ground. You put your forehead down on the pole and spun around the pole as fast as you could several times. Then you tried to return to the starting point as fast as you could. The intent was to get you dizzy and thus make it harder for you to return. We would laugh at people trying to walk or run straight forward. It was impossible. The direction became more zigzag. Sometimes people even fell, probably due to them laughing at the same time.

REACTION

Have you ever come up behind a person to scare them as a prank? I have. The last time I did it was about 30(!) years ago. The reaction was so surprisingly intense that I thought he would have a heart attack. He was warming up on a stationary bike at 6am when I sneaked in to gently tap both sides of his waist as an affectionate "good morning." That gesture quickly turned into a "bad morning." He literally jumped off the bike and ran over to the nearest bench to safety, looking like he had seen a ghost. His overreaction scared the heck out of me to the point where I have not scared anyone in 30 years - I learned my lesson early on in my fitness career. Nevertheless, his fast reaction really impressed me.

Having quick reflexes helps you get out of compromised situations. You have probably experienced, at some point in your life, people bumping into you. If their speed is slow, you're most likely all right, but if they come around the corner at full force and you happen to be distracted at the moment, there may very likely be a collision. Somebody may end up falling and getting hurt. First of all, always be alert, especially around corners. Treat it like a driving incident. If you always prepare yourself by expecting cars coming around a corner with low or no visibility, your reaction will be so much faster if a car actually shows up.

Cautiously practice the Dynamic Drills below to improve your physical reaction. You can do it on your own or you can have somebody else call out "Change Direction" when you least expect it. More creatively, you can record your voice saying different cues intermittently for a minute. Make sure the pauses in between the "orders" vary in length- sometimes short and sometimes long. It's easy to anticipate. Here we go. Get Ready, Get Set, Go!

1. Walk as fast forward as you safely can. Suddenly say "Change" out loud and change to walking backwards as fast as you safely can. Suddenly say "Change" and change directions again. Repeat this about 5 times.

2. Walk as fast side to side as you safely can. Suddenly say "Change" out loud and change to walk side to side as fast as you safely can in opposite directions. Suddenly say "Change" and change directions again. Repeat this about 5 times.

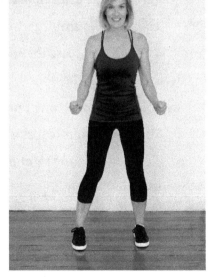

3. Rotate as fast as you safely can in a small circle. Suddenly say "Change" out loud and rotate in opposite directions. Suddenly say "Change" and change directions again. Repeat this about 5 times (or less if you get too dizzy).

You probably recognize this drill is similar to the Dynamic Drill for speed. I'm keeping it simple so you can do more practicing and less reading. This is just to give you samples of different ways to move that you have forgotten over the years. It's all about awakening that body of yours and bringing back those skills to feel more secure.

COORDINATION

A common definition or expression is, "The ability to chew gum and walk at the same time." If you're afraid of feeling clumsy, no worries, you're not alone. We all can work more on our coordination. Get ready to revisit your skills of moving your feet, not only fast and with great reaction, but also with coordination. Wow, I'm asking a lot of you. Yep, I care about the safety of your body and so should you.

You need to be able to move your feet fast. That takes speed, reaction, and coordination. Falls usually start with tripping and not being able to move the feet fast enough to prevent the full-blown fall. That can have devastating consequences.

During these drills, make sure you pick up your feet to avoid tripping. Keep more weight on the front part of the feet to feel you're moving more lightly and softly. When you increase the speed, it will be easier to move the feet faster keeping the heels slightly off the floor.

1. Step out and in with one foot at a time:
   a. Stand with your feet close together.
   b. Take a step to the right putting your weight on your right leg.
   c. Return the right foot.
   d. Take a step to the left putting your weight on your left leg.
   e. Return the left foot.
   f. Repeat a-e as you gradually increase the speed until you can't move your feet any faster safely. Pick up those feet to avoid tripping.

2. Step out and in alternating feet:

   a. Stand with your feet close together.

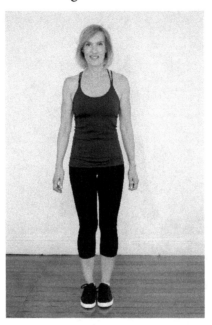

   b. Step out with your right foot.

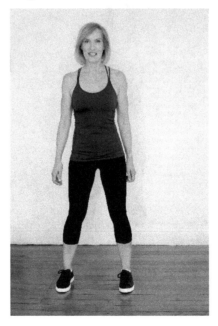

c. Step out with your left foot.

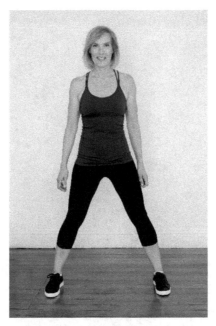

d. Step in with your right foot (return).

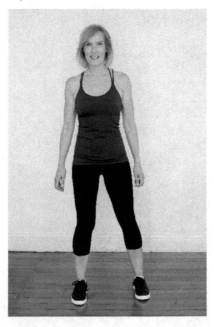

e. Step in with your left foot (return).

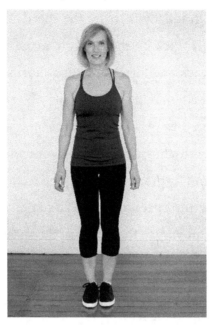

f. Repeat a-e as you gradually increase the speed until you can't move your feet any faster safely. Pick up those feet to avoid tripping. Take a break. You should be huffing and puffing a little bit.

3. Step out and in alternating feet moving forward:

a. Repeat the drill#2 above from a-e.

b. When you have the rhythm, start moving your whole body forward, keeping the out and in movement of the feet.

c. Gradually increase the speed of the feet stepping in and out. Don't increase the speed moving forward. Just the speed of the feet moving side to side. Stop after about 25 feet.

4. Step out and in alternating feet moving backwards:

a. Repeat drill #3 going backwards.

5. Short steps back and forth:

a. Stand with your feet hip-width apart.

b. Take half a step back with the right foot.

c. Take half a step back with the left foot.

d. Take half a step forward with the right foot.

e. Take half a step forward with the left foot.

f. Repeat a-e as you gradually increase the speed until you can't move your feet any faster safely. Pick up those feet to avoid tripping. You're basically moving your feet back and forward, taking short steps.

6. Short steps back and forth moving to the right:

a. Repeat drill #5 from a-e.

b. When you have the rhythm, start moving your whole body to the right side keeping the back and forth movement of the feet.

c. Gradually increase the speed of the feet stepping back and forth. Don't increase the speed moving to the side. Just the speed of the feet moving back and forth. Stop after about 25 feet.

7. Short steps back and forth moving to the left:

a. Repeat drill #6 going to the left.

Do you feel more agile? Agility is the ability to increase and decrease speed, to have control over your movements, to be flexible enough to move in different ways, to be able to change directions quickly at any time with a flow, and good posture.

Some of my clients don't understand why we are doing some of the Dynamic Drills, such as running around cones like football players. We are here to do strength training. Yes, but strength is just one part of your physical health. The way I work out clients 50+ is based on 28 years of experience and unless they move away or pass away, I have a pretty great track record of keeping clients. Some of them have been with me for over 20 years.

At Nordic Body, we add Dynamic Drills as part of the warmup before a workout. It's all about increasing the body temperature, preparing the body to move prior to loading it in the Strength Training segment, and to decrease risks of injuries. If you haven't tried out the Dynamic Drills, let's do some now to get you warmed up prior to some fun and easy Strength Training Exercises. Let's have some fun!

CHECK-IN# 6: MOVE DYNAMICALLY WITHOUT FEAR

Moving the body in different and new challenging ways is great for both the body and the brain. Try out the various Nordic Body Dynamic Drills: Body Awareness, Balance, Speed, Reaction, and Coordination. Pick **one** as a warmup prior to a workout.

1. Which Nordic Body Dynamic Drills are easy for you?

   _____

   Why?_____

   _____

2. Which Nordic Body Dynamic Drills are challenging for you? Why?

   _____

   Why?_____

   _____

3. How long can you stand on one leg? Stand safely on one leg and count slowly or better yet use a timer. Write down the time for the right leg and then the left leg.

   Right Leg_____ Left Leg _____

Did you improve since Chapter One? Use the results from your "stand on one leg" test as your baseline. Check in weekly. There should be some improvement unless you haven't practiced. Practice makes a master. Best way to compare is to use a timer instead of counting. It's more specific.

"Believe you can and
you're halfway there."
~**Theodore Roosevelt**

CHAPTER 7:

Strong is the New Sexy!

Your mindset is stronger, you've put on your C.A.P. and rebooted, and prepared your body for more challenging movement with Dynamic Drills. Now let's get empowered! Think Jane Fonda - look at how she still moves with such confidence, continues to work as an actress, and is driven to make a difference in this world at age 82. Think Queen Elizabeth II - the longest reigning monarch in the world is going strong at age 92. Think Harry Belafonte - he is active in political and social causes at age 91 and appears in movies. Getting older has never looked so good.

A stereotypical depiction of an older person shows them hunched over with bad posture, walking slowly, even shuffling, and looking down at their feet making sure they don't fall. A younger person is most likely to be depicted as walking with a powerful stride, bubbling with life, and showing off an empowering posture. We can still do that as we age - if we are lucky enough to have a functioning body. **The secret is strength!**

Constantly fighting gravity to not bend over into a bad posture, and to not bend your knees, leaving your feet to shuffle, requires muscle strength and body awareness. Your muscles dress your frame, your skeleton. Keeping the muscles strong and flexible will keep your joints stable with good mobility so you can walk around with a youthful, sexy, and empowering stride.

Strength training includes exercises that stress your muscles when working against resistance like your own body weight, resistance bands, free weights, or machines. For example, you use your own body weight as resistance when you do a push-up.

The benefits of strength for both your skeletal muscles and your skeletal bones have been mentioned earlier. However, understanding and retaining this information is so important for your health that I made a brief bullet point list for you to check in with whenever you question why you are doing those darn push-ups, squats, and planks.

5 Benefits from Strength Training

1. Increased metabolism
2. Increased muscle strength
3. Increased bone strength
4. Decreased body fat
5. Prevention of chronic pain

Not a list you could argue against, right? Only positive effects for a longer happier life. Let's break these benefits down in more detail.

Benefit #1: Increased Metabolism

You are your strongest between the ages of 20-30. Muscle mass decreases approximately 3–8% per decade after the age of 30, and this rate of decline is even higher after the age of 60. Muscles are the basis of your metabolism, so if your muscles decrease, your metabolism will also decrease. The solution is to do strength training two times a week to increase your metabolism.

Benefit #2: Increased Muscle Strength

Even if you are past age 30 and you didn't maintain your muscle mass, there is still good news - you can increase your muscular strength at any age - even at 90! Shortly after beginning a strength training program, you will find that daily tasks like picking up grocery bags out of the car seem much easier. This translates into your personal life on many levels. You can stay independent much longer as you age if you can maintain your strength. I see it all the time with my clients.

Benefit #3: Increased Bone Strength

According to the National Institute of Health (NIH), our bones are the strongest at age 18 (if you're a woman) and at age 20 (if you're a man). Once you hit 30, your bones start to get weaker. According to WebMD, about 50% of women 50 and older will have an osteoporosis-related fracture in their lifetime. But by *stressing your bones through strength training, you can increase bone density, reduce the risk of developing osteoporosis, and decrease the risk of bone fractures.

*Muscles attach on bones with tendons. Tendons are the muscles' anchors. Muscles move bones. For example, when the bicep muscle shortens, it brings up the lower arm, looking like a bicep curl. If I place a 3lb weight in my hand, I can do this for hours. But if I grab a 15lb weight, I may be able to do 15 reps until the muscle fatigues. And that's the key word – fatigue! *You have to go to fatigue.* Bones are living tissue. They will get stimulated when you fatigue the muscle. That's how you stress the bones with strength training.

Benefit #4: Decrease Body Fat

As you age, you naturally gain fat. Life is not fair in that women's fat storage actually increases more so than it does in men. Expect to naturally gain between 1 and 3 percent fat for every 10 years after age 20. Don't despair – there is good news! Building muscle helps to burn calories more effectively. The more muscles and less fat you have, the higher your metabolism will be. When you get on the scale, it says only one number. That number **doesn't tell you how much of that is LEAN body weight and how much is FAT body weight.** Lean body weight includes muscles, organs, bones, skin, water, etc. Things we all need to have, right? Yes, we do need some fat as well.

According to Kari Hartel, a Registered Dietitian, optimal health for **men** this range is **10-25%,** and for **women** it's **18-30%**. The goal is the same for men and women; to keep the lean muscle mass high and to keep the body fat mass low.

Lean muscle mass naturally diminishes with age. This goes hand-in-hand with gaining fat. If you don't do anything to replace the lean muscle you lose over time, you'll increase the percentage of fat in your body. **Strength training can help you preserve and enhance your muscle mass at any age.**

My client Marilyn started to work out in her mid-seventies. After just a few months, she started to get compliments from people seeing her muscle definition. It's never too late to start strength training. Just make sure you are consistent. According to a Danish study, <u>it takes just two weeks of physical inactivity for those who are physically fit to lose a significant amount of their muscle strength</u>.

Benefit #5: Prevent Chronic Pain and Decrease Risk of Injury

Improving muscle strength decreases the risk of falling and other related injuries. Developing strong bones and muscles can help to reduce the severity of falls. Increased strength will also allow your body to be more resistant to injuries, and general aches and pains.

Let's focus on a common pain – **low back pain**. According to a blog by *Stenosis Spinal,* low back pain affects almost everybody (80% of adults) at some point and it is the most common cause of disability in Americans under the age of 45. One reason you may experience low back pain is due to bad posture. How is that possible? Imagine a person with bad posture. The back is rounded, placing the head in a compromised forward position. The adult head weighs about 10-11 lbs. The weight of the head is constantly being pulled forward by gravity, resulting in a tug of war with the back muscles, which are endlessly fighting to bring the head back to its optimal position - on top of the shoulders. In that ideal spot, the back muscles can be more normal and more relaxed. If you strengthen the core, the buttock muscles, and the upper back muscles, you will have created a strong defense. This will keep you from giving in to gravity. **According to the Mayo clinic, strength training can reduce the signs and symptoms of many chronic conditions, such as back pain.**

9 Strength Training Exercises and 3 Different Levels to Choose From

Now that you know some of the MANY values of strength training, let's get busy to reap those necessary benefits to age successfully. Put your C.A.P. on (Chapter 3) and please remember to always practice **proper form**.

I have chosen 9 exercises that do not require any equipment so you can start right away. All the exercises are available on video at https://nordicbody.com/wakeup. I highly recommend watching those at least the first time so you can hear my precise instructions. Then you can use the photos in this book as reference next time you work out.

How Do I Warm Up?

Apply everything you have learned in this book so far to stay injury free. Before starting the nine strength training exercises, put your C.A.P. on and warm up with trigger release/correct/load plus some Dynamic Drills. Spend 10-15 minutes all together.

1. **Put your C.A.P. on** (Chapter Three) - Activate the core, align the joints, and apply good posture.

2. **Reboot Your Body** (release/correct/load) (Chapter Five) - Foam roll as many muscles as possible and see if an area needs more attention. Let's say that the right buttock muscle has tons of knots. Continue with a piriformis static stretch for 30 seconds followed by a bridge for 30 seconds to correct the muscle. Finish with a single leg bridge to load the right buttock without experiencing pain.

3. **Choose one of the Dynamic Drills** (Chapter Six) – Try, for example, the *Body Awareness Drill.* Go through all the joints from ankle to neck to see how everything feels and moves.

What Level Should I Do?

Start with Level 1 for the first set. If some of the Level 1 exercises are too easy, try Level 2 during the second set. If they are still too easy, try Level 3 for the third set. If you haven't done anything in years, it may be a good idea to stay with Level 1 and only do one set the first time. If there are any exercises that are causing you pain, stop! Don't do that exercise. When you join the *Nordic Body Monthly or Annual Membership Online,* we provide modifications. Upgrade to the next level wisely. If you have proper form, good technique, and can do 20 reps, or 60 seconds if it's an isometric exercise, then you can test the next level of difficulty. Maybe even mix the two different levels at first. For example, try some push-ups with knees off the floor (level 3) and if you can only do a few then return to being on your knees (level 2) for the rest of the repetitions. Eventually you can do all 20 push-ups with knees off the floor. Level 1 usually serves as a base for Levels 2 and 3. In the videos, I explain it thoroughly, so make sure you listen and watch it at least the first time. You may use Level 1 as a warm-up set the first time you do all the exercises of each month. It's a mixed bag of what you may do. You may never need Level 1 after that.

How Do I Establish a Pain-Free Range of Motion?

Every time you do an exercise in the first set, do five "warmup" repetitions to test the range of motion in your joints. Start with a small range of motion. Hold the end position for 2 counts then return to the starting position. If that is pain free, you can gradually increase the range of motion after each rep. If you experience pain, return to the range of motion that did not cause pain. This may vary from day to day, so always explore to find YOUR body's optimal range of motion. If any range of motion causes pain, try isometric. That means no movement. Just get into the proper pain-free position and hold it.

How Many Repetitions Should I Do?

After the five "warmup" repetitions, move into the "workout" repetitions. The goal is to go to fatigue with proper technique. Quality before quantity. When you do movements like a push up, aim for 20 reps before you up to the next level of difficulty. When you do isometric work like a side plank, build up to 60 seconds before you move to the next level. You do want to go to fatigue to get that beneficial stress on the bones, remember?

What Pace Do I Keep?

After you have done your 5 "warmup" reps to find the pain-free range of motion, then use some **power** (faster pace) to return to the start position of the exercise, **pause**, then lower yourself **slowly** (resist) with control to the end position. There should be 3 phases in a movement when you perform your "workout" repetitions.

1. Fast (power)
2. Pause
3. Slow (resist/control)

If the fast phase causes you pain, what do you do? Either stop or try a slow pace in this phase as well.

There are some exceptions when you do not apply the three phases; for example, any isometric exercises like the isometric side plank. There is no movement when you do isometric exercises. You just hold the position. In addition, the three phases do not apply to exercises like the "Crab and Crab Walk."

How Do I Perform the Exercise?

If you have watched the videos, you should have gotten enough instructions on how to perform each exercise at the three different levels. After that, use the photos. Most exercises will have a START position and an END position. That means you go back and forth between the two positions. Each time you come to an end position, you have finished a repetition. Mimic the photos as much as possible and aim for your best performance.

When Do I Breathe?

The breathing is crucial. Exhale in the power phase (away from gravity) and inhale in the slow phase (towards gravity). If there's no start and end position, that means you hold (isometric) the position in the photo. It's common to hold your breath as well. Don't do that. Keep breathing with rhythm.

Connect Body and Mind

Working out is even more important now than when you were in your twenties. Use your wisdom and awareness when you do specific exercises. It will polish your mental focus and increase your motivation. Get into your body, feel your body, feel how the body is getting stronger. Be grateful for your body. Feel empowered when you can do something longer, heavier, and with higher intensity. Feel how that strength translates into your mental and emotional state. Strengthen your mindset while working out. It is not just about looking good - it is about feeling empowered. How do you feel when you say, "I am building this machine (your body) to last forever so I can live a fulfilling life until my last breath. I am going to make a difference in my own life as well as in other people's lives." Pretty powerful feeling! Be efficient and strengthen the body AND mind by adding some positive affirmations while performing the strength training exercises.

So much to think about? Yes, it takes a lot of awareness to do movements correctly to avoid any unnecessary injuries. We don't want to work out like a 20-30-year-old who is in it for only burning as many calories as possible and may not have felt any warning signals yet to prioritize technique. Instead, we want to work out with wisdom and honor our bodies. If there are aches and pains, we need to respect our bodies and modify an exercise. This is longevity training to keep that machine of yours going strong as long as possible. We are going to live much longer whether we want it or not. Strength training will ensure you live that life with as much quality as possible.

Photos of the 9 Strength Training Exercises (3 Levels)

#1: WIDE PUSH UPS

LEVEL 1: WALL

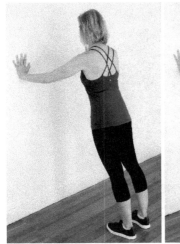 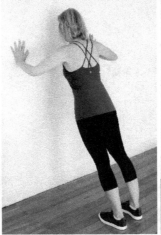 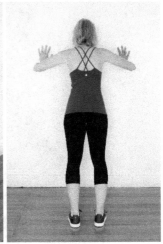

START   END   Proper Position!

LEVEL 2: KNEES

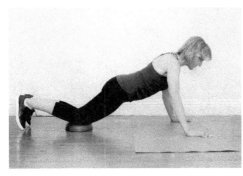 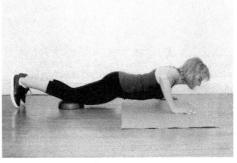

START   END

LEVEL 3: FULL

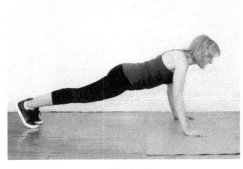 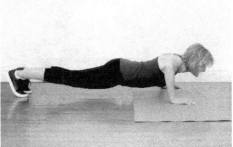

START   END

#2: SPLIT SQUATS

LEVEL 1: WITH SUPPORT (POLES)

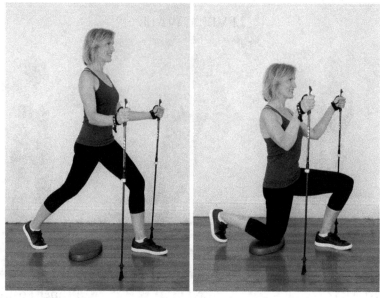

START   END

LEVEL 2: WITHOUT SUPPORT

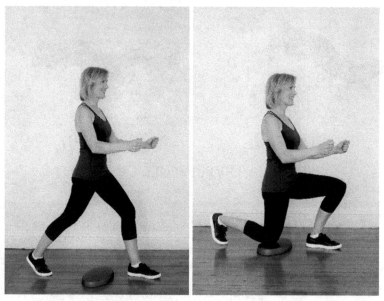

START   END

LEVEL 3: JUMPS

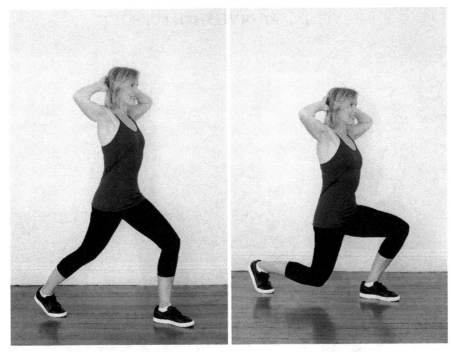

START   DOWN

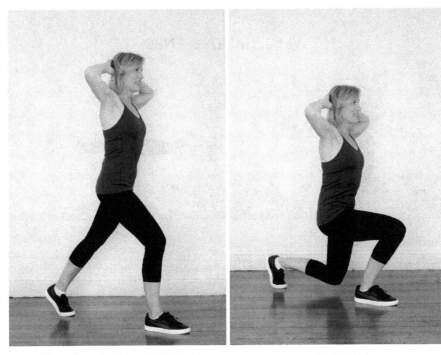

JUMP TO CHANGE LEGS   DOWN

#3: QUADRUPED

LEVEL 1: STANDING WITH SUPPORT

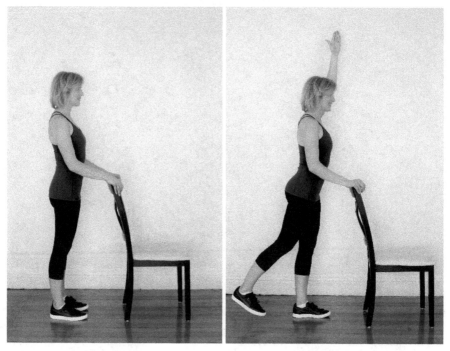

START   END

LEVEL 2: HANDS & KNEES

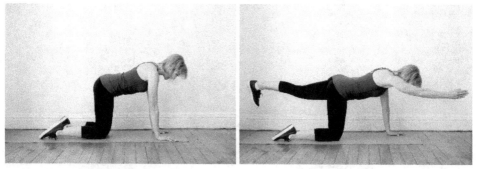

START   END

LEVEL 3: MOVEMENT SIDEWAYS

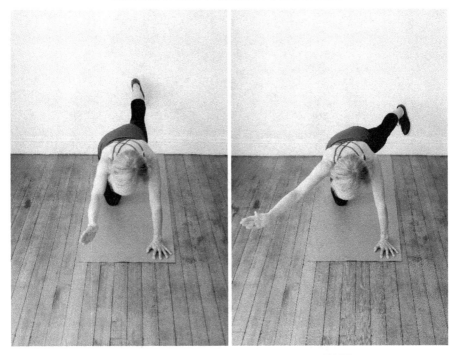

START   END

#4: SIDE LUNGE

LEVEL 1: FEET IN THE SAME PLACE

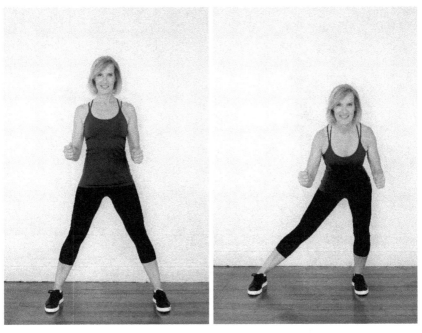

START   END

LEVEL 2: STEP OUT TO THE SIDE

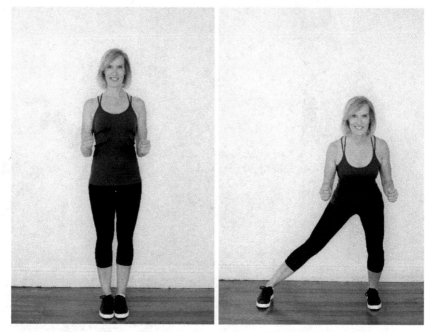

START　　　　　　　　END

LEVEL 3: ADD BALANCE

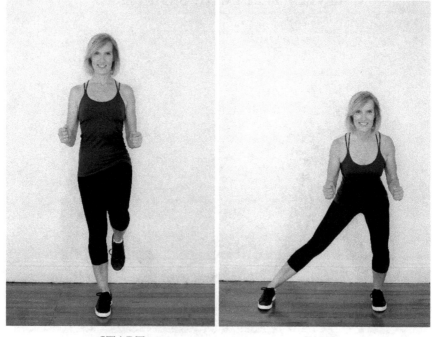

START　　　　　　　　END

#5: OVERHEAD

LEVEL 1: CHAIR – DOWN AND UP

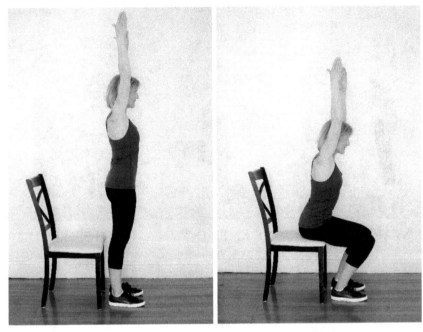

START   END

LEVEL 2: SQUATS – DOWN AND UP

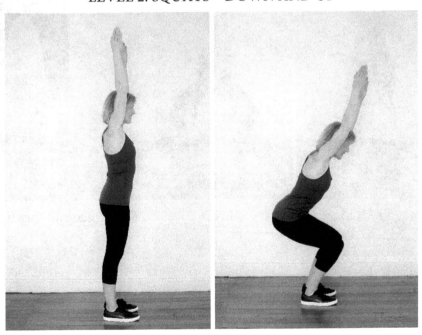

START   END

LEVEL 3: KNEEL DOWN AND UP

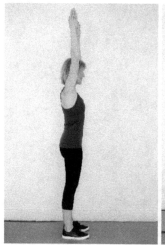 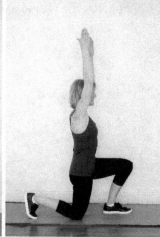 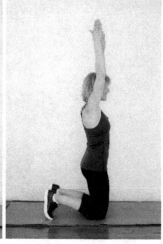

START   ONE KNEE DOWN   BOTH KNEES DOWN

> REVERSE

#6: PLIE

LEVEL 1: WITH SUPPORT

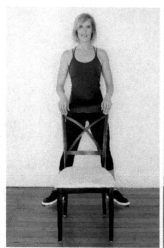 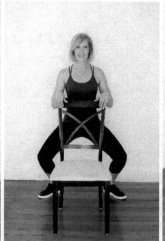 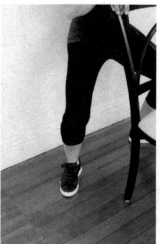

START   END   Keep knee and toes lined up!

LEVEL 2: WITHOUT SUPPORT

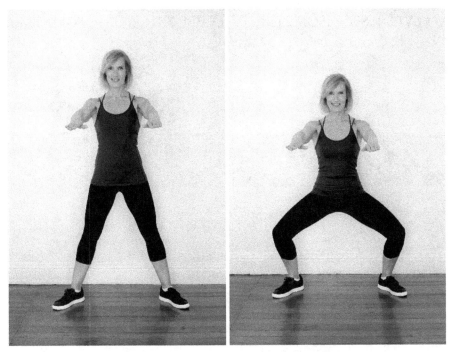

START   END

LEVEL 3: WITH CALF RAISE

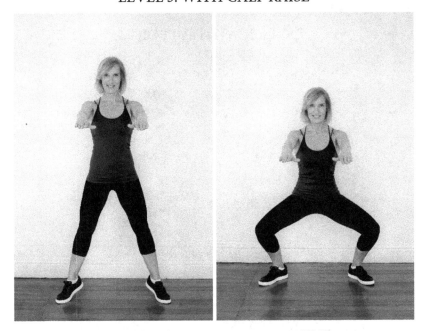

START ON TOES   END

#7: CRAB

LEVEL 1: SIT – ISOMETRIC   LEVEL 2: HIPS UP – ISOMETRIC

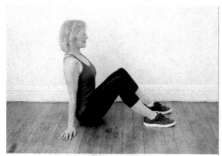 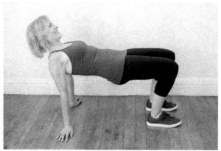

LEVEL 3: CRAB WALK

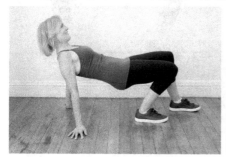 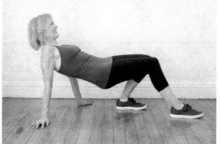

#8: POWER CALF RAISES

LEVEL 1: WITH SUPPORT

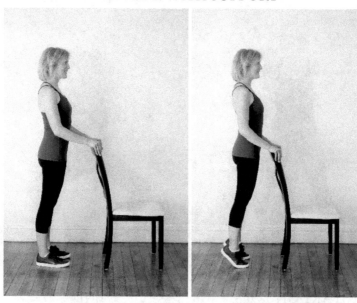

START   END ON TOES

LEVEL 2: WITHOUT SUPPORT

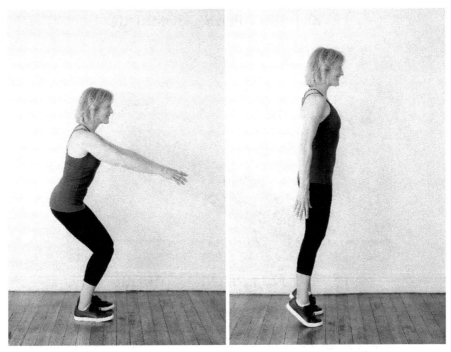

START   END ON TOES

LEVEL 3: JUMP

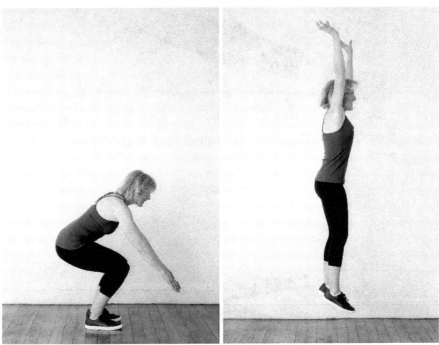

START   END – JUMP

#9: SIDE PLANK

LEVEL 1: HALF PLANK ISOMETRIC

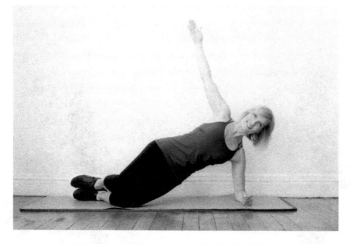

LEVEL 2: FULL PLANK ISOMETRIC

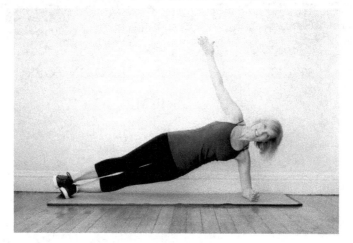

LEVEL 3: FULL PLANK + LEG LIFT ISOMETRIC

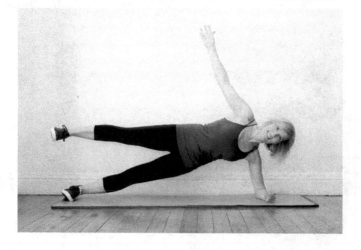

CONGRATULATIONS! YOU DID IT!

Congratulations, you just finished 9 strength training exercises. How do you feel? Keeping my fingers crossed you answered, "Empowered!" A lot of you are scared of doing strength training exercises because you are afraid of getting injured or building up too bulky muscles. A bodybuilder has bulky muscles because they work with such heavy weight that they only can perform the exercise 4-6 times. You will be working with much lower resistance and your muscles will not get bulky.

Are all of my clients injury free? No. However, I believe that they would be more injured if they didn't work out and they would definitely not feel as great. I spend 2-3 hours with each client per week. During the rest of the hours, when my clients are on their own, there are numerous situations that can get them injured. Some people wake up with pain due to how they sleep. Some people get injured from playing golf since they may only swing to one side 5000 times every year. Every time you move your body without awareness you can be prone to injure yourself.

As a personal fitness trainer, my priority is to get my clients stronger without getting injured. The key is body awareness and feedback. I'm big on asking my clients every time I see them how they felt from the last workout. If there's anything that did not feel great, we change or modify the exercise. It requires that they are aware of their bodies.

A lot of us cut off the communication with our bodies from the head down. When we get injured, we have no understanding of how it happened because we take the body for granted to move us pain free from one point to another. Through the rigor and detail of the system I prescribe in my training, you can be a Fitness Detective along with me. Together we can pinpoint the pain, exactly where it hurts and how much, through slow, cautious awareness. All I ask is you promise me you will add strength training twice a week to your schedule. Also, consider joining the community online for accountability.

CHECK-IN#7: STRONG IS THE NEW SEXY!

Empowered and motivated to get strong? Wonderful! I'm thrilled to see the benefits of doing strength training hit home. What are three benefits that gave you that "aha moment" and motivation to commit to doing the 9 strength training exercises? Write the three benefits down and use them as a motivation especially when you try to talk yourself out of exercising.

1. _____

_____

_____

_____

2. _____

_____

_____

_____

3. _____

_____

_____

_____

Elaine Wittert - THE 5TH DECADE

When the youngest and last of my three children left for college, it hit me hard. A nasty slip-and-fall accident around that same time, that took almost six months to recover from, didn't make my life any easier. I couldn't walk, I couldn't drive, I couldn't work, and now with my son gone, I couldn't even parent. Everything that had previously defined me: being physically able, being a social worker, and being a mom had been taken away from me all at once. I felt useless and alone and felt myself slipping into a depression.

To cheer me up, my two sisters invited me to join them on a "get certified in scuba diving" vacation in the Caribbean. I thought they were crazy, but I was curious to try something new. At fifty-five, I learned to dive! To my great surprise I loved it, and when I returned to California, I discovered there were many beautiful places to dive right here in my "back yard." I realized my setback was actually an opportunity to reinvent myself. I received further scuba training, joined a local dive club, and over the next year completed more than 100 dives! I wanted to use my new skill to give back to my community, so I applied to be a volunteer diver at a local aquarium. I had to pass a rigorous skills test to prove I was fit to be on the dive team. It was one of the most physically challenging things I've ever done – but I passed the first time! Now, every weekend I get to dive in a beautiful aquarium while educating visitors about the ocean environment and the importance of protecting it. I have also discovered that being underwater is extremely therapeutic and helps me decompress from the everyday stress from my job as a social worker in a cancer center.

My new hobby inspired me to get further in shape by doing strength training, aerobic exercise, and changing my eating habits (I lost 25 lbs.) Scuba diving is something I'm passionate about, so I'm motivated to keep my body strong and healthy for as long as I can. Malin came into my life to teach me how to correct my muscular imbalances through strength training. In addition, she always encourages a healthy balance of emotional and physical fitness, and I certainly feel I have found that balance. Getting in shape to look good is often not enough motivation to make healthy changes, but being fit enough to carry heavy scuba diving equipment - now that is a motivation that doesn't need explanation. Be strong or struggle! At 56, I can honestly say I have never felt or looked better.

I often like to say I filled my empty nest with water - you can fill yours with anything you like. The goal in sharing my story is to encourage other empty-nesters, especially moms, to embrace this time in your life. It's hard to realize our kids don't need us forever (they do) but fifty is the new thirty and it's never too late to reinvent yourself. Take up that hobby you never had time for, volunteer for a favorite cause, or finally focus on your health and get fit.

~Elaine Wittert (age 56) Santa Monica, CA

"Love the life you live. Live the life you love."

~Bob Marley

CHAPTER 8:

Love Your Heart

Your heart pumps life into your body. How often do you stop to think about that during the day? The first thing I do waking up in the mornings is to put both my hands on my heart and say, "Thank you for today." Your heart and its whole system of vessels (cardiovascular system) circulates blood throughout the body to provide every cell with oxygen and essential nutrients to sustain life. It is in your utmost interest to prioritize the health of your heart. Give it some love. How do we take care of and love our hearts? One way is to do aerobic exercise, which is any type of cardiovascular conditioning (aka: "cardio") including activities like brisk walking, running, cycling, swimming, or cross-country skiing.

Walking and Nordic Walking are the aerobic exercise activities we are going to focus on in this chapter. In addition, you'll learn how to walk correctly to stay injury free, how to vary the walks to make them more fun, and of course all the benefits from walking that will keep you motivated to walk. Fortunately, walking is not only good for your heart, but it is also the most enjoyable form of exercise. Everyone who is fortunate enough to be able to use their legs and can walk outdoors in a beautiful setting probably agree with me. You don't need any equipment; you can do it anywhere and anytime of the year.

As I'm writing this book, we are actually in the midst of the 2020 Coronavirus pandemic. The whole globe is on lockdown with "Safer at Home" restrictions to keep the virus from spreading. In the USA, people are allowed to take neighborhood walks, ride bikes, and go to the park only with their close tribe. Life is quite surreal, like an ongoing *Outbreak* movie from 1995 with Dustin Hoffman and Rene Russo. Families and friends are taking time together more than ever to enjoy the outside spaces. It took a pandemic to get people moving their bodies out from behind their desks!

While much could have been done differently in the government to prepare for such a disaster, one fact remains certain - to be healthy is the best weapon to fight the virus. Having a strong immune system can conquer almost anything, especially having a strong heart. Yes, we know today (March 2020) that the virus's main target is the lungs, but the lungs and heart are very connected. They work together to make sure the body has the oxygen-rich blood it needs to function properly. Oxygen is life!

How does the cycle of life work? The left side of the heart receives freshly-oxygenated blood from the lungs and pumps it out via arteries (blood vessels) to every living cell in your body for it to operate optimally. Your cells use oxygen to make energy and to stay alive. Without oxygen, the cells die, and your organs stop functioning. If the heart does not receive enough oxygen, you can have a heart attack. If the brain does not receive enough oxygen, you can have a stroke.

After the blood has transported oxygen and nutrients, it returns back home via veins (blood vessels), this time to the right side of the heart. The blood has lost all its oxygen and needs to pay a visit to the lungs for cleaning and re-oxygenation. After that process, the lungs can once again deliver oxygenated blood to the heart and the whole staying alive journey starts all over again.

A deconditioned heart has to work harder to get oxygenated blood through the body. According to the American Heart Association, it appears elderly people with coronary heart disease or hypertension are more likely to be infected and to develop more severe symptoms. As said by the Kaiser Family Foundation, almost half of Americans ages 55 to 64 have at least one pre-existing medical condition that exacerbates their risk.

This is wakeup call time! Let's see how walking **briskly** on a regular basis can easily be your solution. Look at all the benefits below to the problem we just talked about. Rise up to this occasion and make a difference in your life - make it a healthier one. Yes, as we age, we are more susceptible to viruses and such, but we can prepare and build a stronger defense system. Don't you agree it's better to enter a battle with a strong body and mind instead of a weak one?

Benefits From a Regular Brisk Walking Routine

- Improves your *cardiovascular fitness
- Strengthens your heart
- Boosts your immune function
- Extends your life
- Lowers your risk for heart disease, stroke, and diabetes
- Improves blood flow and circulation
- Manages high blood pressure
- Improves cholesterol levels
- Controls blood sugar levels
- Maintains leg muscle strength and bone density
- Eases joint pain
- Burns more calories
- Improves your sleep and mood
- Boosts your energy levels - less fatigue/more stamina
- Improves brain function
- Improves balance and coordination
- Gives your mind a break

The cardiovascular system basically includes the heart, blood, and blood vessels

Can you see how walking benefits your heart health? Yes, very exciting! Now I need to point out that these are not the benefits from a stroll in the park. You need to walk briskly. This is a Walking Workout compared to the Active Lifestyle we talked about in Chapter 4, where you didn't have to change into your workout clothes. To reap all the benefits from the above list, we must take the pace up a notch. I highly recommend you put your workout gear on, including some comfortable walking sneakers. If you already walk 10,000 steps a day, then good for you! Now, honestly, how intense are those steps? Is it like on your "day off" pace, which I also call an "active rest" day? Is it window shopping pace? Is it walking your dog pace with stops and starts? Don't get me wrong, any movement is wonderful. However, we are here now to do a Walking Workout, which requires us to focus only on walking for 20-30 minutes, or longer if you have the stamina.

According to the Centers for Disease Control and Prevention (CDC), 80 percent of adult Americans do not get the recommended amounts of exercise each week. Ages 65 and older are least likely to engage in physical activity.

Let's Walk Correctly to Prevent Injuries

People look at me with amusement when I tell them I am going to observe their walks. If there are some incorrect patterns, they laugh when I say I will help correct them. Every person who is able to walk thinks he or she can walk. Yes, a person can go from point A to point B. But how efficient and how pain free is that walk? When your foot lands, it has so many options to move (or not move) due to muscle strength, stability, and flexibility in the whole body. When you apply all your body weight on that poor foot seconds later, your ankle joint had better get all the support it needs from the correct muscles to carry your weight. Clients stop laughing, especially if aches and pains disappear, as they rediscover their bodies and become aware of how they walk.

The practices below may seem like overkill, but when you slow down and really pay attention to all the mechanisms of your walk, you will change the way you walk all the time, not just aerobically. Practice one step at a time of the ten steps below as you walk around indoors or outdoors. See how it feels and be aware of your walk next time, whether you go for a stroll or a walking workout.

1. Land With the Heel to Clear the Floor

When you take a step with the foot, you want to make sure you land with the heel first; more specifically, with the center of the heel first. If you land more on the inside or outside of the heel, it may have an impact up the line to the knees, hips, and the rest of the body. Having the ability to clear the floor is crucial to prevent falling. I'm sure you have seen people shuffle. They don't land with the heel. It requires strength in the front of the lower leg and flexibility in the ankle. While watching TV, you can keep the front of the lower calves strong by bringing all ten toes up (keep heels on the floor) and pause then lower them slowly. Repeat that 10-20 times. If you simultaneously feel a stretch in the back of the calves, you're doing it correctly.

2. Roll Onto the Rest of the Foot

After you land with the heel, continue to roll onto the rest of the foot. You can practice this rolling movement by first standing still and rocking back and forth from heel to toes like a rocking chair. Then try walking backwards. Though it will be reversed from toe to heel, it is sometimes easier to feel the rolling movement when you walk backwards. Please be careful. Make sure you have a clear path behind you. Then shift gears and walk forward to apply the rolling movement from heel to toes.

It is fairly easy to hear feet that don't roll, especially with shoes on when you're going downhill. There is a slapping sound. Feet that roll are almost soundless. Are your feet noisy or quiet? If you are prone to sore shins, the slapping of the feet could be one cause.

Avoid the arch collapse. Though there is a slight pronation (rolling inward) during the landing of the foot, the arch should not roll in too much or collapse. You need to have a strong foundation to land on in order to hold up the rest of the body. If the arch collapses, maybe the knee and the hip will follow. If untreated, this instability through the joints each time you take a step can eventually lead to injuries.

At the end of this phase you are standing solely on one single leg. This is why balance training is so important. Walking with confidence requires balance. If you don't feel secure, return to Chapter 6 and practice balance and other Dynamic Drills.

3. Heel Lift

As you roll onto the ball of the foot (base of the toes), the heel comes off the ground. If you previously did the rocking-back-and-forth movement, you may have experienced the sensation. During a calf-raise exercise, that's exactly what you practice - lifting the heels off the ground. This action requires strength and flexibility in the calf muscles and feet as well as mobility in the ankle joint. When the heel of one foot starts lifting off the ground, the opposite foot starts landing. You now have more or less support from both feet. That's why people with a limp hurry back to feel the support of the other foot on the ground as well. It's just too painful for them to linger on one foot only. Pay attention to any pain while walking. Bring your experience to a health and fitness professional to help you correct any muscular imbalances you may have.

4. Push Off to Increase Speed

Use the ball of the foot to push off. This push-off action propels the body forward. Walk around and feel how you push off with the base of the toes. To be more precise, with the base of the big toe and the second toe. You should feel that you increase the speed when you push off to walk forward.

5. Connect With the Buttocks

At the same time you push off with the ball of the foot, you activate the very bottom of the buttock. That is singular. Tighten only one buttock. Feel the connection between push-off action of the ball of the foot and the activation of the buttock of the same leg. Yes, you can help shape your buttocks while walking. A wonderful perk!

6. Lean Slightly Forward as One Unit

As you walk, make sure you lean slightly forward **as one unit** from your heels to your head. Always keep that core activated to avoid any bending in the waist or rounding of the back as you lean forward. The leaning forward feels almost as if you are falling forward. If you don't like that image, instead imagine a big magnet that is pulling you forward. The weight should be on the balls of the feet. Walk around and see how it feels to lean forward as one unit. Does it feel as if you are increasing your speed? If so, you are doing it correctly.

When we walk uphill, we have a natural way of leaning forward. Keep that feeling when you walk on flat surfaces. Just watch out for any bending in the waist or upper back.

7. Arm and Leg Rhythm

Start walking with a clear path in front of you. After a few steps, glance down so you can see your left arm swinging forward. Next, observe which foot lands at the same time. Yes, the right foot lands at the same time the left arm swings forward. Basically, the left arm meets the right leg, and the right arm meets the left leg. This is the natural walking rhythm, and most people don't even think about it—it just happens naturally. If you can't see it, exaggerate the arm swings to match the pace of the legs. If it gets you out of rhythm, then stop to shake it off, and start walking again. For fun, experience walking with the same arm and leg at the same time. That should feel really strange. If you don't feel the difference, have somebody videotape your arm and leg movements. Seeing it with your own eyes can be very helpful for making adjustments.

8. Even Arm Swing

When you have the arm and leg rhythm down, make sure the arm swing is even. In other words, you should swing the arm as much forward as you swing it backward. This is hard to see on yourself unless somebody videotapes you from the side.

Another solution to increase your awareness is to take two chairs with high back supports. Place them about three feet apart with the back supports facing each other. Place yourself in the middle of the chairs. Do your arm swing alternating left and right. When you swing your arms, the hands should reach the back supports of both chairs equally. Most clients I observe have an easy time swinging forward. When I ask them to increase the backswing to make it more even, the forward swing increases even more so they are still not in balance. This arm swing in between two chairs should be very helpful. Apply this awareness next time you're out walking.

9. Slight Rib Cage Rotation

When you did the arm swing exercise with the chairs, you may have noticed a slight rotation in your upper body. That is correct. A lot of people walk around with very stiff backs. The arm swing should be initiated from the trunk with a slight rib cage rotation. This will loosen up your back muscles. It's worth a try!
Let's practice in front of a mirror.

- Stand still with feet hip-width apart and place your hands on the sides of the rib cage just below the chest.
- Keep your head and hips straight as you softly turn the rib cage from right to left with the help of your hands.
- Feel the twist (rotation) happening around the solar plexus, where the axis of the rotation takes place.
- Try maintaining this twisting movement as you release the hands.
- Start walking and add this slight rotation to your walk.
- Don't slow down but keep a regular pace.

This soft, upper-body rotation matches the lower-body rotation. The upper-body rotation results in movement of the shoulders, and the lower-body rotation results in movement of the hips. A common mistake is to move the shoulders by themselves without initiating the slight rotation. The initiation of the rotation is in the axis. This means that if you focus on initiating the slight rotation in the solar plexus (located in the center of the torso above the navel), the shoulders and hips have no choice but to move.

10. Straight Arm Swing

When you add a slight rotation of the torso (step 9), it's very common to start crossing the arms in front of you. That's incorrect. The rotation happens only in the ribcage. The arms maintain a straight arm swing forward and back.

Before leaving the arm swing, I need to mention a tip about your hands. Though your hands are at the end of the arms, their position is crucial for your posture. Are the palms of your hands facing the thighs or turned so the front of the hand is facing forward? Walk behind a person and see if you can see the palms of their hands while walking. That means that their shoulders are internally rotated. This separates their shoulder blades and promotes a rounded back. Bad posture! It's such a small thing to keep the palms facing your thighs while swinging your arms, but it sure makes a huge difference in your posture. Now, your shoulder blades are not fixed during the arms swing. They move, but by bringing awareness to your hand position, they can move more efficiently.

By exploring all the ten steps you should be walking as if you are on top of the world!

Nordic Walking - An Upgrade of Your Regular Walk

Now that you have mastered your own walking technique, it will be easy to **add Nordic Walking poles** to intensify your walk and get into shape even faster. Everyone wants to take a miracle pill and get fit instantly. Well, here's your miracle pill - Nordic Walking!

The first time I tried Nordic Walking was on the sand in Santa Monica in early 2002. I got very upset because I thought my heart rate monitor was broken. It went up high, as if I was running -140 beats per minute! Granted, I was walking on soft sand, but still, c'mon, I was just walking! When I realized my heart rate monitor worked perfectly well, I was sold on Nordic Walking. Having been a runner all my life, I had started to feel some aches and pains in my hip and ankle in my late thirties.

Working out with poles was a welcome solution. I got just as good of an aerobic workout as running, but with low impact and my upper body got a workout too! What's there not to like? It's an awesome activity.

Additional Benefits from Nordic Walking Compared to Regular Walking

Nordic Walking is an enhancement of regular walking. All the benefits from walking were mentioned earlier in this chapter. The benefits below are **additional** advantages from **adding poles** to your walking workout *based on* using a correct pole technique.

- Burns 20 to 46 percent more calories.
    - Basic Nordic Walking burns on average 20% more calories.
    - Fitness Nordic Walking burns about 46% more calories.
- Increases upper-body strength, especially uphill.
- Increases heart rate by 5 to 30 beats per minute.
- Takes pressure off the ankle, knee, and hip joints, especially downhill.
- Decreases neck and shoulder pain and stiffness.
- Increases upper-body mobility.
- Feels like less of an effort even though the body works harder (burns more calories with less effort).
- Improves balance and stability, making it safer to walk.
- Improves gait and coordination.
- Improves core stability and posture.
- Creates a meditative and calming effect.

Nordic Walking will not only increase the intensity of your walking workout and get your heart into better shape faster, but it is also a fun activity to do with a group of people. Since you can use any surface, you can meet up at somebody's house in the city, at a park, by the beach, or at a trail in the local mountains. What can be better than doing something healthy with a group of friends? As we age, we tend to isolate and feel lonely. Nordic Walking can be the perfect solution to socialize while improving the health of your heart. Take advantage of Nordic Walking by creating a meditative effect. What better way to repeat your positive affirmations during a walk with your poles? Every time you touch the ground with your feet and the "feet" of your poles, you connect with Mother Earth. You feel more grounded in your body and mind,

What Equipment Do I Need for Nordic Walking?

You only need to purchase a pair of Nordic Walking poles. Everything else is the same as when you do your walking workout. I suggest investing in a water belt around your waist with space for a phone, keys, ID-card, credit card, and some cash. You need to be hands-free when Nordic Walking since your hands will be busy holding onto the poles. Visit our website for more information on the Nordic Walking poles I recommend https://nordicbody.com/.

Time to Learn Basic Nordic Walking

If you still don't understand why people use poles while walking, do the following simple test. You need only a chair, a table, and two arms. Sit down on a chair by a table and place your left hand (in a fist) on the table. Place your right hand (flat) on your abdomen. Press the left fist down into the table and release. Repeat this action of press and release. What happens in the abdomen as you do this action? Yes, it activates. Move the right hand around to the chest, back, and back of the arms. The same thing happens with those muscles. This is why you use poles in Nordic walking: to engage the muscles in the upper body. Every time you apply pressure to the pole in the planting phase, the upper body muscles awaken.

If you have ordered poles but they haven't arrived yet, practice the regular walking techniques. That will prepare you better for using the poles. If you have the poles, time to take them for a spin.

1. Find the Natural Walking Rhythm With the Pole

To practice finding the natural walking rhythm, find a big open area that has no obstacles ahead of you. Stand still with poles strapped in. Relax your arms and shoulders. Let the arms just hang heavily at your sides. Open the hands to make them even more relaxed. If you have strapless poles, just barely hold on to the grip. Forget for a moment that you have poles hanging from your hands. Now, start walking as if you were just going for a leisurely stroll. While the poles are dragging on the ground, the arms are swinging to match the leg rhythm. Don't think – just walk. After about 25 feet of walking this

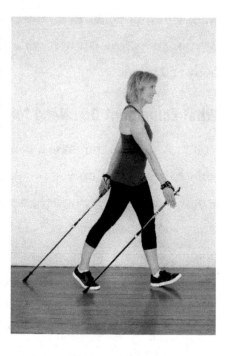

way, glance down at the right arm. Observe it as it swings forward. Check which foot lands as you swing the right arm forward. It should be the left one. Opposite arm meets opposite leg – that's the walking rhythm.

2. Plant in a Handshake Position

Once you have the natural walking rhythm, increase the height of the arm swing forward. You should start feeling the tip of the pole catch the ground. That is the crucial moment! The second you feel that traction, grab the grip of the pole and plant the pole firmly on the ground. All fingers should be wrapped around the grip. Remember to take advantage of the pushing through the strap as well.

Make sure the arm is in a handshake position when you plant the pole. It's common

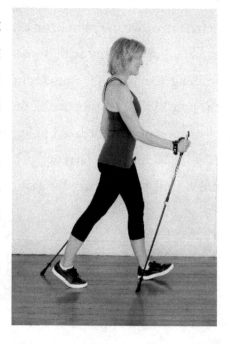

for people to glue their elbows to the waist. They miss out on a big part of the back muscle getting engaged. Make sure you free the elbows from the waist and place the arm in a handshake position instead.

You should feel how the arm and other muscles of the upper body are engaged. Make sure you give the grip a good squeeze as you plant the pole. If you only tap, you won't engage as many muscles. Walk around and compare the feelings of planting the pole firmly to barely planting the pole. The great thing about a snugly fit strap is that it should be used to transfer the power. This way, your knuckles won't turn white from pressing down on the grip.

3. Push the Hand Back to the Hip

As you plant the pole, keep applying that firm pressure as you push back and down on the pole. This is the action that will propel the body forward, and this is why you plant the pole at an angle and not vertically. You don't want to move up to the sky; you want to move forward. This is the easiest one to describe, but it requires the most of your effort. While some people have strong backs and arms and can thus push farther back, others will have to practice more. It's a good motivation, though, because it will strengthen and shape the back as well as the 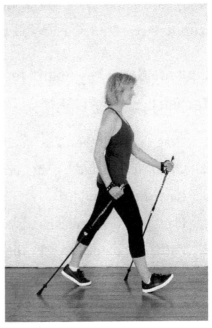 triceps. We women especially love the backs of the arms shaped! Start Nordic Walking!

When you feel you have pushed as far back as you can, soften the grip a little before you return to planting the pole. With a snug strap, it should still feel that you are one with the pole. It should not feel like you are about to lose the pole when you soften the grip. If so, stop to tighten the strap. It will take some practice to get the coordination of the squeeze as you plant and the slight release at the end of the pushing phase.

Once you can maneuver this, your muscles will be very happy. They will go from tension to relaxation. If you walk around with constantly tensed muscles, you will become fatigued and your muscles will be sore. Practice this coordination and your muscles will learn to stay more relaxed.

Voila, you're Nordic Walking! To ensure you are not dragging the poles, walk briefly on asphalt without the paws (aka: rubber tips at the bottom of the poles). If you hear a clicking sound once as you plant the pole, you are doing it correctly. If you hear a dragging sound, you are still dragging the poles. You can easily correct this by Nordic Walking temporarily without paws on asphalt (or any hard surfaces) until you are able to hear only one clicking sound.

Here Are Some Key Points for Building Your Basic Nordic Walking Technique:

1. Drag the poles ONLY to get into the rhythm.
2. Opposite arm and leg rhythm.
3. Keep the pole angled.
4. Plant pole firmly in a handshake position.
5. Push back to the hip using both the grip and the strap.
6. Soften the grip by the hip.
7. Return to planting; pole is airborne.
8. Do not drag the poles - it's not part of the finished technique.

Anyone at any age can do Basic Nordic Walking. If it's easier for you to learn Basic Nordic Walking from watching videos, go to https://nordicbody.com/wakeup

For me, I need to add different terrains, like hills or sand, to get my heart rate up while doing the Basic technique. That's why I created the complete Nordic Walking Program. I teach various techniques, from Regular Walking to more advanced options like Fitness Nordic Walking, which is the technique I mainly use when I go Nordic Walking.

What Do I Do Now?

You have polished your walking techniques, you have your poles and know basic Nordic Walking, you have your walking workout clothes, including shoes and hopefully a water belt so you can drink water while walking or Nordic Walking. Now what? A lot of customers ask me **how long** they should walk, **how often,** and at **what pace.** Treat walking and Nordic Walking as any aerobic exercise. The American College of Sports Medicine (ACSM) defines aerobic exercise as any activity that uses large muscle groups, can be maintained continuously, and is rhythmic in nature. Examples of aerobic exercise include brisk walking, cycling, dancing, hiking, jogging/long distance running, cross-country skiing, and swimming. Centers for Disease Control and Prevention (CDC) recommends adults get at least 150 minutes (for example: **30 minutes x 5 days**) of **moderate-intensity aerobic exercise** each week or 75 minutes (about 20 minutes x 4 days) of vigorous-intensity activity, or a combination of both to improve fitness and reduce risk of illness and disease.

Five Ways to Vary Your Walking Workouts

Variation is key! Just like we vary the strength training exercises, we need to vary the aerobic exercises. The body strives for balance and loves when we keep doing the same thing day in and day out. It gets very comfortable and knows exactly what to expect. It doesn't have to use any extra energy (calories) to figure out anything new. However, to avoid boredom, to burn more calories, and to decrease the risk of injuries, I recommend you vary your aerobic exercises too. One example can be to change the activity itself from walking to Nordic Walking. You can also change other variables like route/program, time, pace, and terrain to surprise the body in a good way. Here are five suggestions to spice up your walking workouts.

1. **Route/Program**

Raise your hand if you're guilty of always walking the same route. No worries. I can be guilty of that sometimes too. I have a perfect 30-45 minute route in my neighborhood in Santa Monica. One way to vary it is to reverse it. Do your best to come up with other routes. Maybe walk with friends to check out their favorite walk. If you walk on a treadmill, it is easy to change programs.

2. **Time**

This can easily be changed, and it goes hand in hand with the next variable intensity. If you just have 20 minutes to walk, make it vigorous. With this intensity, you should only be able to say a few words. If you have 30 minutes or more, make it moderate. With this intensity, you should be able to talk but not sing your favorite song. If you can, bump it up.

3. **Intensity**

You can either keep the same intensity for the whole walking workout or you can change it up by doing intervals. This is one of my favorites. I love changing intensity by doing intervals. Interval training can be performed in many ways, but the general idea is to alternate periods of relatively intense exercise with recovery, either low-intensity exercise or rest. The length of the intervals can be anywhere from 20 seconds to 3 minutes. If you are new to trying out different intensities, it may feel too hard to do vigorous intensity. Instead, choose a longer interval at a lower intensity than vigorous. If it's difficult for you to use a timer to keep track of the intervals, then you can choose a landmark instead. For example, you walk fast for one block and then slow for the next block. You walk fast up a hill and then slow back down again. Be creative, there are no rules.

4. **Terrain**

Varying terrains can really make a difference, even for your bone density. Walking is weight-bearing and thus we can maintain bone density on flat surfaces. It takes more impact, like running and jumping, to build bones. However, walking up many stairs and up steep hills can also build bones and even muscles. If you have access to soft sand, try that terrain. It's quite a challenge.

5. Techniques

Early in this chapter, you reviewed basic regular walking to make sure you are using a technique that is as optimal as possible to stay injury free and to help you intensify your walk. If walking is not enough for you to get your heart rate up, try Nordic Walking. It takes fitness walking to a new level by adding poles to produce an incredible full-body workout.

Taking care of your heart is essential for many reasons that you have learned throughout this chapter. Schedule your walking workouts in your weekly calendar just like you do any other appointments. The busier you get the more important it is to take care of your heart to reduce stress. Don't skimp on your walks to free up your time. Be more efficient and arrange walking workout dates with friends and family so everyone can benefit from both socializing while building more energy and endurance.

CHECK-IN #8: LOVE YOUR HEART

It is nice to hear somebody say, "I love you," but it is even nicer when somebody shows by their actions that they love you. Don't just say "I'm going to work out tomorrow." Take action. Go for a walking workout now and show your heart you love it! What are three things you are going to do right now to get your heart into better shape?

1. _____

_____

_____

_____

2. _____

_____

_____

_____

3. _____

_____

_____

_____

Bo Svensson – THE 7TH DECADE

Throughout my life, I've always enjoyed staying physically active, but I noticed it decreased more and more as I was aging. Every time I would say with determination, "This Monday I am going to start working out 3 times a week," it would never come to fruition due to lack of motivation. As I explored what would motivate me, it hit me – enter a challenging competition! This would definitely force me to get into good shape. Otherwise, it would be too brutal to do the competition. The better shape I would be in, the easier and more enjoyable the competition would be, right? After some research, I decided to enter the world's largest cross-country ski race in Sweden – Vasaloppet. It was a perfect choice since it was 12 months out and it would give me plenty of time to train for this 90 km (56 miles) race in the snow. The preparation also included the weather that would be quite cold, but invigorating, with stunning scenery in the "Alps" of northern Sweden. Another reason I chose a cross-country skiing race is that it has a reasonably mild impact on the body unless you end up falling too many times at high speed down the hills.

As I started to train at age 68, I realized that the skiing technique was different than the one I had learned 40 years ago. However, I decided to keep the good old way that I was used to instead of having to re-learn something new. The inspiration to work out increased and it was a great feeling. I knew the race would take approximately 8-11 hours for an amateur like myself and the notion of getting in as great shape as possible to have an enjoyable experience was a magical motivation. Unfortunately, on race day, I was pulled out of the race for not completing the first 50 km under 7 hours – my time was 7:03! Unbelievably frustrating! Three minutes less and I could have continued! Have you ever been angry with mountains? Well, I was because the mountains had zapped my energy and cost me those three minutes. I felt I had the capacity to complete the race the following year. To show the mountains I could do it, I made a date with them that summer and walked the same path as the race. It was a great mental exercise that increased my confidence.

Luckily, at this time my little sister, Malin Svensson, decided to jump in to help me. With new energy, new skiing technique, and in better shape due to her valuable coaching tips, I was able to finish Vasaloppet the following year when I turned 70! What a way to start a new decade! Full of possibilities! Now I do the Vasaloppet every year and I'm back to being physically active as I'm aging - I feel so good! Who knows, maybe I'll do the Nordenskiold Loppet, which takes place north of the Polar circle and is 200 km (124 miles) in snow in super cold weather. After all, I will always be a Viking regardless of my age. You can be one too. Find something (event, competition etc.) that would motivate you to stay physically active. It works!

~Bo Svensson 72, Stockholm, Sweden

"It's fun to do
the impossible."
~**Walt Disney**

CHAPTER 9:

The Wonderful World of Stretching

Yay, you finally get to stretch! This is your reward for all your hard work. Spoiler alert: you know I'm not just going to give you ONE stretch though. No, I'm going to show you FOUR different ways to stretch. Most people just say stretch. They don't specify what kind of stretch they are doing. There's more than just one way to stretch those muscles to loosen them up and to increase the range of motion around the joint.

If you have a tight muscle, do you go straight to a static stretch? Meaning you hold the stretch for 30 seconds? You're not alone if you choose static stretching as the only way you stretch. Don't get me wrong, I use static stretching a lot. But, guess what? There are other ways that will actually be a better choice depending on the scenario. Sometimes static stretching shouldn't be your go-to way. Sometimes trigger release, active, or dynamic stretching should be the preferred choice. In this chapter, you'll become familiar with four different ways to stretch. You'll learn how, when, and why to do each particular stretch. A whole new world of stretching is available to you. Get ready to adjust your mind to new ways of stretching!

Why Do I Need to Stretch?

Do you skimp on stretching to save time? Please don't! Stretching is as important as the workout itself. As we age, our muscles tighten and the range of motion in the joints can decrease. This limitation may be due to either joint replacements, arthritis, an injury, or just simply tight muscles. That restriction will limit you when you try to sit down, which requires your ankles, knees, and hips to bend. Have you seen people crash land on a couch or even a chair without any control? They may not have the flexibility of the muscles to allow the optimal range of motion in the knee to occur. They may also lack the strength in their legs, especially the buttocks. Stretching can help improve flexibility. Better flexibility will improve your performance in physical activities and decrease your risk of injuries by helping your joints move through their full range of motion. The ability of a muscle to stretch is called flexibility and the ability of a joint to move is called mobility.

Being Too Flexible Can Be Bad

Think Cirque du Soleil. Those acrobats get into unimaginable positions as if they had no bones in their bodies. While we all may be in awe during their performances, I'm sure their bodies will be regretting it as they age. **It is just as dangerous to have muscles be too flexible as it is to have muscles that are too tight**. You want to rely on your joints for stability. You don't want to experience the scary feeling of them giving in. Muscles, tendons, and ligaments help to create support around the joint. If you are prone to be very flexible, be careful with lengthening the muscles past their optimal length. Focus more on strengthening the muscles around the joint to provide stability. For example, our shoulders are the most mobile joint, but also the most unstable one. It is the easiest joint to dislocate. Make sure you keep the muscles around the shoulder joint strong. Keep the shoulder joints flexible enough to move it in all directions, but if you are too flexible, be careful stretching the muscles around the joint past its normal length.

The same caution should be applied to elbows and knees. Some people are too flexible around those joints, causing hyperextension. This forces the joint to bend the wrong way and puts a lot of stress on those joint structures. In addition, being too flexible around the knees can create bad posture. For example, hyperextension of the knees (hamstring muscles stretched to the max without firming up the front thigh muscles) will create havoc on your posture.

Let's travel up the body and see what happens from the knees to the head. Hyperextended knees push the hips forward, resulting in the back forced to lean back, and in turn forcing the head to push forward, fighting gravity to prevent falling backwards. It only takes one tiny adjustment to straighten everything back to normal and that is to soften the knee joint and activate the quads. It's amazing to see how one little movement like that changes the whole posture from bad to good. So being too flexible is not always great for your joints. *If that's you, focus more on strengthening your muscles than stretching them.*

Why We Have Joints

Imagine not having any joints. You wouldn't be able to brush your teeth, lean forward to tuck in your kids at night, or walk upstairs. The way your body is able to move is due to the movement of the joints and how the muscles work around the joint. For example: take your biceps (front of the upper arm) and triceps (back of the upper arm) muscles. When the bicep muscles contract and shorten, the tricep muscles relax and lengthen. That teamwork between the biceps and the triceps makes it possible for you to bend your elbow. Too much tightness due to arthritis, injuries, or a sedentary lifestyle can make the joints stiff.

Maintaining the optimal length of muscles is crucial for natural movement. Muscular imbalances occur when muscles are too tight or too weak on one side. Strengthening weak muscles is taken care of by doing strength training and paying attention to which side is weaker and stronger. The tightness of the muscles is solved by various ways of stretching.

The Four Different Ways to Stretch

Throughout this book, you've gotten a taste of the four different ways to stretch. Trigger Release followed by specific Static Stretching stretches are covered in Chapter Four. We used Active Stretching during the Body Awareness Drill in

Chapter Six, and for the five warm-up repetitions of a strength training exercises in Chapter Seven. The split squat exercise in Chapter Seven is an example of Dynamic Stretching. So, I have provided enough information for you to do all the stretches correctly. Now we're diving deeper.

During two of the four stretches below, you will hold the position for a length of time. This is a great opportunity to integrate the body and mind connection. Are you struggling to find time to do your positive affirmations? Now is a great time! Anytime you work with your body, take time to really connect with the muscles. If you only go through the motion to just get through the stretch, you are missing out on some real treasures. Bringing awareness to your muscles as you stretch is like going deeper inward. Open up the communication and you will better understand your body and be able to better take care of it. Concentrate on the muscles being stretched. Connect with the muscle. You'll get a better stretch. Be aware of where you feel the stretch and which side is tighter and needs more attention. Breathe!

While you're doing any of the stretches below, be grateful for your body and praise yourself. Feed your body and brain with positive affirmations. Connect your body and your mind. Take a deep breath. Let it go. Surrender. Feel free. Feel the lightness. Feel the freedom of the movement of your body. Ahhhh…. it's a wonderful feeling.

1. Trigger Release

Trigger release followed by static stretching is part of The Nordic Body Reboot Program. However, you can also use trigger release by itself. When you pick up other literature, you may find this same concept called by a fancier word, such as self-myofascial release, or just simply self-massage. Who doesn't want a massage? Getting a massage from yourself can sometimes be even better because you get to hang out where those sore knots need it the most.

What: Apply gentle force to an adhesion ("knot") for 20-60 seconds by using a trigger release tool like a foam roller.

Why: There are specialized receptors inside of tissues that respond to pressure and send out signals through sensory nerves. They respond to forces such as motion, pressure, stretching, and touch. When tension from a foam roller is applied to the muscle, a message for help is sent to the brain, which reacts by sending out an order to the muscles to relax. We trick the brain into helping us relax the muscle - a process called autogenic inhibition. The pressure from the trigger release tool will release the knot 50-70%, changing the elastic muscle fibers from a bundled position (knot) to a straighter alignment in the direction of the muscle or fascia. Those once-knotted muscle fibers can finally become more useful. You have awakened muscle fibers that have been asleep - they can now participate in helping the whole muscle to work and function more properly.

When: Can be used anytime. For example, prior to a workout as part of the warm-up; in combination with the *Nordic Body Reboot Program*; after a workout to prevent soreness. If you're in a rush, do at least the buttock muscles. I roll through the whole body daily prior to my first client of the day. When I do it, it looks like such a flow, so I call it the "Trigger Release Dance."

2. Active Stretching

During the first five repetitions prior to a strength training exercise, I use active stretching as a warm-up. I prepare the muscle for that movement, making sure there are no aches and pains, but also trying to increase the range of motion by stretching the muscle involved.

What: Take the joint gradually to its end range of motion and keep it there for approximately two seconds. Repeat 5 times.

Why: To lengthen (relax) one muscle for the opposing muscle to shorten (contract). It's called reciprocal inhibition and it's a neuromuscular reflex that inhibits opposing muscles during movement. For example: if you contract your elbow flexors (biceps), then your elbow extensors (triceps) are inhibited. Joints are controlled by two opposing sets of muscles, extensors and flexors, which must work in synchrony for smooth movement.

When: Prior to a workout as part of the warm-up to prepare your muscles for activity in the short term.

3. Dynamic Stretching

Athletes use this for warmup. In this book, you will experience it during some of the strength training exercises, for example: the split squat. To make an exercise more difficult, try to go deeper into a full range of motion while executing the exercise. Did you know you were actually also stretching while building strength? Another great motivation to do strength training!

What: Active movements like Active Stretching, but taking the body through the full range of motion smoothly without holding it for any length of time. For example: walking lunges. This can put a high demand on the soft tissues including muscles, tendons, ligaments, fascia, and nerves. The dynamic stretches can be functional and mimic the movement of the activity or sport you're about to perform.

Why: Dynamic stretches are meant to get the body moving. They take your muscles and joints through a full range of motion using reciprocal inhibition to extend the range of motion of the joint.

When: They can be used to help warm up your body before exercising. Unless you're a natural athlete, I would use them instead in your strength training program, since they encourage the max range of motion of the joints. Better to build up the range of motion gradually than go straight for the deepest and lowest position.

4. Static Stretching

This is the way of stretching that most people resort to when something is tight. After this chapter, I hope you know when to use it and why. For example: doing it *prior* to a workout may decrease your performance. However, as with most rules, there are always exceptions if you understand the concept. Below you'll find those *exceptions*. Enjoy!

What: Get into the stretch position. Go to only a mild discomfort. Hold for 30 seconds, but don't hold your breath. Remember to relax, breathe in and out. Every time you breathe out (exhale), feel how the muscle gives in more and more. If you go past mild discomfort you will do yourself a disservice. The muscle will not trust you and thus it will not relax and give in (lengthening) which defeats the purpose of the stretch.

Why: When you hold a low-force stretch for a time, like 30 seconds, it creates alarm in your body. The poor receptors are feeling the built-up tension from the ongoing stretch and send signals to the brain to "send help" to relax the muscle before something bad happens. It is the body's beautiful way of protecting the muscles and tendons to avoid getting injured. Mission accomplished! Once again, we have tricked our brains to allow a further stretch. Static stretching can actually make a difference in the length of the muscle, not just temporarily, but also long-term. That's why it's so powerful when used together with the trigger release. They are a great team helping you correct muscular imbalances in your body. It's never too late!

When: Mainly done post workout to get the normal length returned to muscles or slightly further if needed. Static stretching is also used in combo with trigger release (to get rid of knots) to be able to further lengthen the muscle. Pay attention if one side is always tighter. For example: let's say your right calf muscle is always tighter. Then use static stretching on the right side only prior to the workout for the sole purpose of getting the tighter side to loosen up so it's more equal to the left side. Use it in conjunction with trigger release to get better results.

For the next many pages, you will find tons of examples of different stretching routines to do after a workout or during the day to either wake up better in the morning, get more energy in the afternoon, or get a better night's sleep.

Ten Static Stretches *Indoors* After a Workout

These will be done mainly lying down since most of the time we do strength training exercises indoors and we have easy access to a mat and walls.

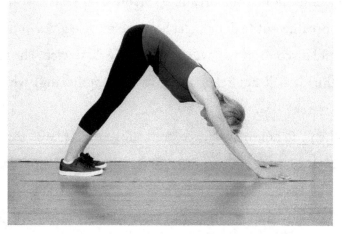

Downward Facing Dog

1. **Downward Facing Dog** on a mat. Come down to all four - hands and knees. Spread your fingers and keep the fingertips curled to reduce the pressure on the wrists. Tuck in your feet - curled. Keep the knees bent as they leave the mat while you're lifting the hips high up toward the ceiling. Keep the heels off the ground and keep pushing the hips up by pushing from the ball of the feet. Keep your hands on the mat while gently moving the chest towards your thighs each time you exhale. Now gently lower the heels to where it feels comfortable. Gently straighten the knees without moving the chest away from the front thighs. Stay there, breathing deeply, connecting with the muscles being stretched. Enjoy the 30 seconds while reciting a positive affirmation.

2. **Back and Shoulders:** Lie down on the floor with feet up 90 degrees on a wall - bring the arms back above your head and let gravity do the stretch for you. Place the arms where they are in a pain-free range.

3. **Piriformis:** With your feet still up 90 degrees on the wall, bring your right foot up across the left knee - arms can be on the floor in a t-position with palms facing up. Move the buttocks either closer to the wall or further away to feel a stretch in the right buttock area. The sacrum (bone between the buttocks)

should be on the floor. After 30 seconds, change legs. If necessary, change the position of the buttocks either further or closer away from the wall to feel the stretch and to keep the sacrum down. Stretch the side that is tighter two times. Remember that next time so you start and finish with the tighter side.

4. **Hip Internal Rotators:** Same position as the prior stretch, but this time place both hands on the inside of the knee and push it away from you. You should feel this stretch more in the front groin/front side of the hip/buttock area. Change sides and pay attention to if one side is tighter. Apply the same formula as the prior stretch.

5. **Hamstrings:** Move your whole body away from the wall so both feet barely touch the wall when the legs are totally straight. Bend both knees. Bring one knee to your chest like you're hugging the knee. Then gently straighten that same leg up to the ceiling keeping your hands just above the back of the knee. Keep the sacrum on the floor. Try to pull the toes down on the leg you're stretching to feel a nice stretch on the calf in addition to the hamstring. If possible, stretch out the leg that is not being stretched on the floor with the toes pointing up and the heel pushing towards the wall. After 30 seconds change legs and repeat. If one side is tighter than the other, you know what to do by now.

6. **Side of Trunk:** Bend both legs, keeping the knees and feet close together. Arms positioned like a T with palms facing up. Gently let the knees fall to the right side, keeping the left shoulder down touching the floor and gently turn the head looking to the left. After 30 seconds, activate the core and return only the left leg first followed by the right. Change sides and repeat.

7. **Inner thighs:** Bend both legs, keeping the knees and feet close together, but the soles of the feet facing each other and touching if possible. Let the knees fall out to either side. Keep the core active to prevent too much arching of the lower back. Can you see if one knee is higher than the other? If not, they may be the same tightness.

8. **Child's Pose:** Roll over to one side and come up on all fours. Gently get into a child's pose by lowering the buttocks towards the heels while leaning forward with the upper body so the forehead almost rests on the mat. If you have ankle

or knee problems, place a cushion behind your butt so you don't sink down too deep and hurt your knees. Test to see if you can straighten the arms out in front of you on the floor. Are the shoulder joints preventing this? If so, keep the elbows bent.

9. **Hip Flexors:** Gently raise the upper body so you're only on your knees. If your knees cannot take the pressure, do a standing hip flexor stretch. If the knees are fine, do a kneeling hip flexor, bring the right foot in front of you flat on the floor with the knee bent 90 degrees. The ankle should be lined up with the knee joint. Tuck the pelvis in and under (flatten the back) and tighten the left buttock to feel a better stretch in the front upper thigh. Hold on for support if needed. Lift and reach your left arm up to the ceiling. After 30 seconds, change sides.

   a. Standing hip flexor: Stand with feet hip-width apart. Hold on to support if needed. Take a long step back with the left leg. Look down to check both feet are looking straight ahead. Tuck the pelvis in and under and tighten the left buttock to feel a better stretch in the left upper thigh. Lift and stretch the left arm to the ceiling. After 30 seconds, change sides. Note: the bonus is you may also feel a stretch in the calves by doing it standing up.

10. **Quads:** If needed, hold on for support when you grab the ankle of your left foot, maintaining great posture, and gently move the left leg so the left knee is pointing straight down to the floor. If you want to feel more of a stretch, tuck the pelvis in and under and tighten the left buttock. After 30 seconds, change sides.

The **Ten Static Stretches *Indoors* After a Workout** are also available on video at https://nordicbody.com/wakeup

In a rush after the workout is over? Here's a quick and dirty one:

1. Downward facing dog
2. Child's pose
3. Kneeling hip flexors

Six Static Stretches *Outdoors* After a Workout

These will be done mainly standing up since we walk and Nordic Walk outdoors and may not have the opportunity to lie down. I'm assuming you have poles to be used for support - if not, just use something else in nature for support.

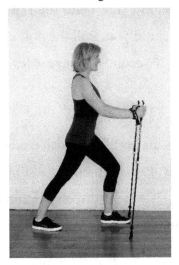

Standing hip flexors with poles

1. **Hip Flexors & Calves:** Standing hip flexors

2. **Back:** Stand hip-width apart. Place both poles as far in front of you as possible. Bend your knees, bend in your waist, straighten your arms as much as possible. Your end position should look like the back is a table. After 30 seconds, pull in the navel and curl up one vertebra at the time until the head comes up last.

3. **Chest & Neck:** Let the arms fall to the sides with palms facing forward. Reach for the ground with the fingertips, and squeeze the shoulder blades together, opening the chest. At the same time, gently turn your head to one side, stay there 10 seconds, return, and turn the head to the other side. Then return and tilt the head with the ear to one shoulder, hang out 10 seconds, and tilt the head to the other side.

4. **Piriformis Standing:** Feet hip-width apart. Take the right foot and place it on top of the left knee. Bend down into a squat position until you feel a stretch in the right buttock. After 30 seconds, change to the other side.

5. **Quads**: Place the poles in a tripod position, holding on with one hand on both pole grips. Grab your left ankle and bring the knee down to look straight down. Feel the stretch in the left quadriceps. After 30 seconds, change sides

6. **Triceps**: Grab one pole with your right hand. Straighten the arm up toward the sky, but place the pole behind you. Bend the right elbow. Take your free left hand and find the pole behind you. Pull the pole down until you feel a stretch in the right triceps. After 30 seconds, change sides.

Stretches on the Go

Having healthy daily routines makes life so much easier. They act as solid pillars in your sometimes-scattered day. Expand them by adding more healthy steps toward a complete healthy lifestyle. The next three stretching routines are mixed with Active and Static stretches, functioning as a check in with your body on how to feel better from the moment you wake up until it's time for bed. Why not add those positive affirmations here as well as you breathe slowly and deeply? Connect your Body and Mind.

1. Morning Routine to Awaken the Body Better

A lot of people feel more pain and stiffness in the mornings when they get up. No wonder - the body hasn't moved for eight hours! Movement lubricates the joints. The fluid is called synovial and is present in the joint capsule. Your car needs oil, right? Well your joints need to be "oiled" too. Next time you feel stiff, think movement and active stretching to lubricate your joints.

Unless you have to rush out of bed to use the restroom first thing, try these fifteen moves to get your body and mind to fully wake up. It sounds like a lot, but it's a wonderful way to start the day off. So worth it. You may not end up doing all fifteen all the time. Choose the ones that help you the most. If anything hurts, do it even more gently and with a smaller range of motion. If it still hurts, don't do the movement.

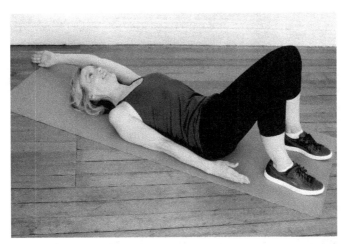

Windmill

1. **Start the day with gratitude**: Lie on your back. Place both your hands on your heart. Take three deep breaths in and out through your nose. As you exhale, say a positive affirmation like "I am grateful for today."

2. **Pelvic tilts**: Gently pull in your navel as you bend the knee and slide one heel on the bed up towards your buttock. Place the foot flat on the bed. Then do the same with the other leg. Place your arms by your side relaxed with palms facing up to the ceiling. Gently pull the shoulders away from your ears. Do five gentle pelvic tilts, holding each position for two counts. (Pelvic tilt is alternating flattening the back to release or gently arching the lower back.) If anything hurts in the lower back, do it even more gently and with a smaller range of motion.

3. **Windmill**: Place your pelvis in neutral. This means your lower back is neither flat nor arched. Lock that position by gently pulling in the navel. Gently bring both arms up to the ceiling, palms facing each other. Make sure you don't lift the arms so high that your shoulder blades are pulled apart. Do a total of ten (five for each side) gentle windmills holding each position for two counts. (Windmill is alternating moving one arm down towards the bed while the other one moves straight back towards your ear.) If anything hurts in the shoulder joints, do it even more gently and with a smaller range of motion.

4. **Bridges:** Place the arms back down on the bed with palms up. Gently tighten the buttocks and gently push the heels down into the bed. Exhale and gently lift the buttocks off the bed. Pause at the top for two counts. Lower the buttocks with control. Repeat five times.

5. **Knee hug:** Grab one knee with both hands and gently move it towards your chest. Hold it for two counts. Gently release. Repeat five times, then switch legs.

6. **Knee extension:** With bent knees and feet flat on the bed, gently lift one knee toward you, keeping the upper leg at 90 degrees. Place two hands behind the knee or just below it. Gently try to straighten the knee by pushing the heel up to the ceiling. Hold it for two counts, then gently return. Repeat five times. Switch legs.

7. **Side to side:** Keep the knees and feet close together, arms positioned like a T, with palms up. Gently lower both knees to one side. Hold it for two counts. Pull in the navel and return both knees. Switch sides. Repeat a total of ten (five to each side).

8. **Spread the toes:** Roll over to one side and come all the way up sitting on the edge of your bed. Scooch back so only the feet and half of the calves are off the bed. Spread all ten toes. Hold them spread for two counts. Then repeat five times.

9. **Heel raises:** Sit on the bed with feet flat on the floor. Lift both heels slowly up as high as possible. Aim to be on the ball of the feet. Hold it for two counts. Slowly return. Repeat five times.

10. **Toe raises:** Walk your feet out about a foot. Pull all ten toes up. Hold that position for two counts. Slowly return. Repeat five times.

11. **Stand/Sit:** Sit on the edge of the bed. Tighten the buttocks. Push the heels into the floor. Place your hands on your lap. Lean forward with your back so the butt comes off the bed. Slowly straighten the legs. Finish by straightening the upper body. Pretend you have a string from the crown of

your head. Pull it up and lengthen your spine. Hold it for two counts. Reverse and SLOWLY sit back down, keeping the weight and focus on the buttocks and heels. Repeat five times.

12. **Balance:** Standing tall, slowly shift the weight over to one leg and fire all the muscles on that side of the body. Feel that side as a solid pillar. Hold that position for two counts. Repeat ten times (five on each side)

13. **Arm swing:** Stand tall and feel the shoulders pulled away from your ears as you lengthen the neck. Fingertips reach for the floor. Gently alternate, swinging the arms straight forward and back from the shoulder joint. This looks like a pendulum from the side. Keep each arm swing position for two counts. Repeat ten times (five one each side).

14. **Heel strike:** Stand tall. Place one heel in front of you with all five toes pulled up. Hold that position for two counts. Alternate changing legs. Repeat ten times (five on each side)

15. **Fully Awake:** You are now ready to walk out into the world. Alternate arms and legs. Landing with the heel to prevent falls. Your body and mind should be fully awake.

2. Mid-day Routine to Stay Alert

Raise your hand if you start drowsing off in the afternoon. Before you grab that caffeine drink, try some of these moves to perk you up. Increase the blood circulation to get more oxygen to the body and the brain. Move the joints to decrease the stiffness. Think good thoughts, especially if the day is not going the way you want it. Change the body, change the mind. Those positive affirmations are perfect in the afternoon to get you into a better mindset, better spirit, and becoming more productive.

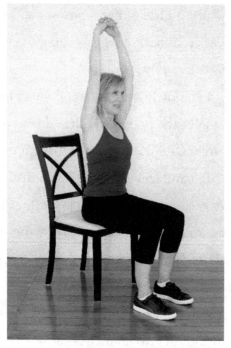

Overhead

1. **Overhead:** Sit in your seat and reach both arms above your head as you exhale. Hold the end position for two counts. Repeat five times.

2. **Back of the arm:** Reach one arm up, bend it. Place the opposite hand on top of the elbow joint. Apply pressure down and slightly back on that elbow. Feel a stretch in that triceps muscle. Hold that position two counts. Release. Repeat five times before switching arms.

3. **Neck Turns:** Sit back in the chair. Scooch back so the buttocks touch the back support. Let the arms hang down the side of the chair. Turn the hands so the palms are facing forward. Reach the fingertips to the floor while pulling the string from the crown of your head up to the ceiling. Retract the shoulder blades. Feel both arms touching the back support equally. Keep that position the whole time. Gently turn your head to one side. Hold it for two counts. Release. Repeat to the other side. Do a total of ten (five on each side).

4. **Neck Tilts:** Same as the previous stretch. Instead of turning your head, you are now tilting the head to one side, ear to shoulder. Hold it for two counts.

Pull in the navel and return the head gently. Repeat to the other side. Do a total of ten (five on each side).

5. **Super Tall:** Stand up, reaching those arms up to the ceiling again, but now you also come up on your toes. Hold the position for two counts. Sit down slowly. Repeat five times.

6. **Balance**: Stand tall. Lift one knee at the same time you lift one arm straight up (windmill). Hold the position for two counts. Alternate knees and arms. Do a total of ten (five on each side).

7. **Hip Flexor & Calf:** Keep your core active. Raise both arms above your head. Take a step forward. Keep that knee slightly bent. The back leg stays straight. Feel a stretch in the calf as well as in the hip flexor of the straight leg. Hold the position two counts. Change legs. Repeat. Do a total of ten (five on each side).

8. **Fold & Unfold:** Stand with feet hip-width apart. Slowly squat down, putting weight on the heels and buttocks. Try to touch the floor with your fingertips. Hold that position for two counts. Curl the spine up one vertebra at a time – head comes up last. At the same time you are curling the spine, you gradually straighten the leg (the legs are doing most of the work to protect the lower back).

9. **Hand Walk:** Same as previous movement, but as you touch the floor with your fingertips, keep walking your hands as far forward you can. The goal is to eventually end up in a pushup position. Hold the end position for two counts. Then gently return back up by bending the knees and getting the heels down on the floor before you curl up the spine using your legs to return to standing. Repeat this whole challenging move five times. If you have lower back problems, proceed with caution!

10. **Quad & Chest:** Stand tall. Gently bend one knee, aiming to kick the butt without arching your back. Hold position for two counts. Alternate legs. Do a total of ten (five on each side).

b. As a bonus, you can add an arm movement: Keep the arms straight out to the sides at shoulder height. Bring the arms together in front until the hands touch with palms facing each other. Return the arms to the starting position and feel the shoulder blades squeeze together. Hold that position for two counts. Repeat five times.

You should feel ready to kick some butts for the rest of the day. Hopefully you will feel rejuvenated and alert to finish the day strong both mentally and physically.

3. Evening Routine to Sleep Better

With all that sitting during the day, we are shorter at the end of the day compared to the morning. Let's do some stretches to lengthen that body of yours before bedtime to reset it. Time to let go of the day, especially if you didn't have a good one. Time to surrender. What happened can't be undone and there is nothing you can do until tomorrow. It is crucial you start and finish the day on a good note. Most of the time we can't do anything productive until the next day, so really try to let go of anything that worries or bothers you. Use some powerful positive affirmations as you are stretching and getting ready for bed. I believe it is important that you start getting ready for bed at least 30 minutes before bedtime by dimming the lights, doing some relaxing stretches, deep breathing, and calming positive affirmations. Give it a try! What do you have to lose? You may even gain some hours of restful sleep so you can better deal with the next day.

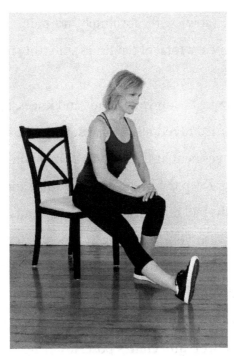

Hamstring and Calf

1. **Hamstring & Calf:** Sit on the edge of a chair. Straighten one leg and keep the heel on the floor with the toes pointing up. Gently pull those toes toward you to feel a stretch in that calf (lower leg). Place both hands on the opposite bent leg. Sit as tall as you can while gently leaning forward with a straight back until you feel a stretch behind your knee, in the hamstring and your calf. Hold it for 30 seconds. Perfect time to recite a positive affirmation. Each time you exhale, feel how the muscle gives in and how your mindset feels lighter. When time is up, use your hands to push yourself back up to make sure the lower back does not do the main work. Change legs and repeat.

2. **Piriformis:** Sit on the edge of a chair. Bring the right foot on top of the left leg. Sit as tall as you can while gently leaning forward with a straight back until you feel a stretch around the buttock area. Hold it for 30 seconds. Switch legs. Repeat.

3. **Cat Cow:** Come down to the floor on a mat or carpet. Be on your hands and knees. Exhale and gently push your upper back toward the ceiling rounding the back letting the head hang relaxed between the arms (cat). When you can't exhale anymore, reverse. Inhale and gently look up, get your chest up and gently

arch the lower back (cow) with absolutely no pain. When you can't inhale anymore, reverse. Repeat a total of ten times smoothly moving to the rhythm of your breath.

4. **Downward facing dog**: Stay on your hands and knees. Spread your fingers and keep the fingertips curled to reduce the pressure on the wrists. Tuck in your feet - curled. Keep the knees bent as they leave the mat while you're lifting the hips high up to the ceiling. Keep the heels off the ground and keep pushing the hips up by pushing from the ball of the feet. Keep your hands on the mat while gently moving the chest toward your thighs each time you exhale. Gently straighten the knees as much as you can without moving the chest away from the front thighs. Gently pedal your feet, alternating lowering one heel at a time. Hold it for two counts then switch feet. Repeat a total of ten times (five on each foot)

5. **Child's pose:** Gently drop into child's pose, lowering the buttocks towards the heels while leaning forward with the upper body so the forehead almost rests on the mat. If you have ankle or knee problems, place a cushion behind your butt so you don't sink down too deep to hurt your knees. Test to see if you can straighten the arms out in front of you on the floor or are the shoulder joints preventing you? If so, keep the elbows bent.

6. **Bridge:** Roll over to your back. Place your feet hip-width apart. Move the feet fairly close to the buttocks - about a foot between heels and buttocks. Arms relaxed by your side with palms facing up, trying to get those thumbs to touch the floor. Shoulders away from your ears and slightly retracted. Do some gentle pelvic tilts to find your neutral spine. Tighten the buttocks and push down on the heels. Exhale and slowly lift up your buttocks from the floor. Stay in the highest position (without straining your neck) and hold it for 30 seconds. Go inward and connect with the working muscles making sure everything works equally. Though the buttocks are working and getting strong, the hip flexors are getting the static stretch. We need them to lengthen after sitting a lot during the day.

7. **Inner thighs:** Keep lying on your back. Bring your soles together and let the knees fall out to the side. You should feel a stretch in the inner thighs. Check in with your lower back. Sometimes it is too arched in this position. Gently tilt the pelvis without flattening the lower back completely. Lift your head to check if one knee is higher or lower. If one is higher, gently put your hand on that inner thigh and press gently down to get a better stretch. Stay here 30 seconds. When time is up, pull in the navel and gently return one leg at a time.

8. **Side:** Keep lying on your back with both legs bent with feet on the ground. Move the knees and feet close together. Arms out like a T with palms facing up. Cross right leg over the left leg. Gently let the knees fall to the left side, keeping the right shoulder down touching the floor and gently turn the head looking to the left. If you want more of a stretch, place your left hand on the right knee leg and gently press down without getting the right shoulder lifting off from the floor. After 30 seconds, activate the core, uncross the right leg, and return it first followed by the left. Change sides and repeat.

9. **Quad:** Roll over on your left side in a fetal position. Grab the right ankle with your right hand and gently bend the right knee until you feel a stretch in the front thigh. The right heel should be closer to the right buttock compared to when you started. Pull in the navel to avoid any lower back pain. Hold the static stretch for 30 seconds. Release. Repeat on the other side.

10. **Spine Lengthening:** The best position to lengthen the spine is to place your legs up on a chair while you are lying on your back. The buttocks need to be super close to that chair, so the knees are 90 degrees (knees lined up with hips). Stay here for a few minutes, focusing on slow deep breathing.

11. Have a wonderful, restful sleep with a taller height.

Hope you have enjoyed the wonderful world of stretching and that you have stretched your mindset as well to try some new ways. This chapter concludes all the movements for the body in this book. Now we are moving into what we need to eat, how we can stay on track and get inspired to upgrade your life to the next level. All while you are feeling empowered to lead a complete healthy lifestyle for the body, brain, and mind.

CHECK-IN #9: WONDERFUL WORLD OF STRETCHING

Now you have the knowledge of the different ways to stretch (trigger release, active, dynamic, and static). Create your favorite list of five or more stretches that you can do during the day. Before working out, after working out, in the morning, afternoon, and before bedtime.

My Favorite Stretching List:

1. _____

2. _____

3. _____

4. _____

5. _____

_____

_____

_____

_____

_____

_____

_____

"I never worry about diets.

The only carrots that interest me are the number you get in a diamond."

~Mae West

CHAPTER 10:

Feed Your Body and Brain

You can't outwork a crappy diet! Even if you work out for an hour a day and get in your daily 10,000 steps by leading an active lifestyle, you will still not feel or look healthy if you do not watch what you eat. For your car to work optimally, you use premium fuel, and some luxurious cars even require super premium fuel. Food is fuel for the human body. More than ever, you have to think about your body as a machine that performs based on how well you take care of it. Treat yourself like a Porsche! Eating healthy has to go along with having a healthy body, brain, and mind This is the single most reason people struggle with getting in shape - resistance to changing their eating habits - which affects all parts of the process. I get fed up (pardon the pun) when people start talking about not only what they ate, but how many calories and how many ounces. To me, that's not very empowering, but more of an obsession, from which I try to stay away. Instead, I believe everything in moderation, especially when it comes to exercising and eating.

Healthy Eating 101

When you hear "healthy eating" do you relate it to weight loss only? Hopefully not. I want to tell you upfront: I am an expert in exercising and getting you strong, not in nutrition and helping you lose weight. Weight loss is a bonus byproduct from participating in my strength training programs. Frankly, focusing on weight loss is not the right mental state. Instead, I choose to focus my clients on what we easily can do - get stronger. In that process, when clients see results, they also get motivated to improve their eating habits. Another reason I don't focus on weight loss in my programs is that the phrase in itself is such an emotional trigger that it screws up people's minds. Emotional eating is outside my expertise and handled beautifully by coaches, who handle these issues. If, on top of struggling with making healthy food choices, you have an emotional trigger to food, I highly recommend you contact a person specializing in that area. For example, a good resource is my friend, a registered dietitian (RD), Robyn L. Goldberg. She is an expert in eating disorders and wrote a book about it called *The Eating Disorder Trap*.

So, what is considered a healthy diet? First and foremost, foods that give your body the nutrients and energy it needs to function properly generally include clean foods (meaning not processed, and organic as much as possible) and plant-based, and includes fresh fruits, fresh vegetables, whole grains, low-fat dairy products, lean proteins, and healthy fats. Experiencing less energy, sleep deprivations, and pain can all be due to nutritional deficiency. The saying, "You are what you eat" is really true.

When I host my Holistic Fitness Retreats, I take it a step further and offer an organic lunch that is also gluten free, sugar free, soy free and dairy free. It's like a detox for many participants. Except for serving eggs, sometimes our lunch is also a great vegan option. Often participants have not treated themselves to food this clean and fresh in a while, and they get to experience how different they feel in the midst of making their bodies stronger.

According to Max Lugavere and Paul Grewal MD (authors of the book *Genius Foods*), the best way of eating for an optimally-performing brain is consuming a diet that is high in nutrient-dense foods. he ten genius foods in their book are extra-virgin olive oil, avocados, blueberries, dark chocolate, eggs, grass-fed beef, dark leafy greens, broccoli, wild salmon, and almonds. They recommend avoiding foods that cause hormonal dysregulation, oxidative stress, and inflammation like processed oils and grain products.

Already you can see there are some conflicts. Eat grains, don't eat grains. Eat eggs, don't eat eggs. Eat meat, don't eat meat. Every expert will give you their version of what is healthy. Focus on what they all agree on. Research and gather information about foods they don't agree on. Then make the choices that work best for you and your body.

Added Sugar Causes Chronic Inflammation in Your Body

The guidelines I will give you here are based on my own experience. I was lucky enough to be brought up in a home where we ate healthy and it has become a natural way for me to live. However, my family, especially my mom, are known for having a sweet tooth. Because we exercise, lead an active lifestyle, and generally eat healthy, we are all in good shape. Would it be better to not consume the added sugar? Absolutely! I took that extra step and got rid of my sweet tooth six months after I turned 50. Before that, I would have one cookie a day while I enjoyed my afternoon tea, but I had to go down to Starbucks to buy it every day. If I had a whole package of them conveniently at home, they would be gone in one day. I know I have little to no self-control with sugary foods in my house. Know yourself and figure out a way for you to avoid any traps. In addition, I kept Saturday as my "junk food day" which for me meant I had sweets in addition to my healthy main meals (breakfast, lunch, dinner). What happened six months after I turned 50 was a colonoscopy, which is a recommended test here in the USA when you turn 50. The result was great, but the preparation for the procedure was not a fun experience with trying to empty everything in your colon so the intestines were nice and clean. While coming home from the successful colonoscopy procedure, I walked down to Starbucks for my daily cookie and tea. As I stood there in line looking at the large 300 calorie chocolate chip cookie, it didn't look appealing to me at all, so I didn't buy it to my shocked surprise. The same thing happened the next day, the next week, and the next month. Wow! What had happened? My close friends and family could not believe it when I said, "No, thank you" to a chocolate chip cookie. Now, eight years later, I still hardly ever eat anything with added sugar like chocolate, ice-cream, candy, cookies, or cakes. I suspect what happened was that my system was so super clean that my body and mind said, "Wait a minute. You have just spent half a day cleansing your system and now you're going to put that junk into your super clean intestines?" I really don't know any other explanation. Anyway, I was certainly not going to force myself back to having a sweet tooth and that's how fortunate I have been for eight years. Due to that, I stay away from anything that has chocolate flavor, like protein shakes, no matter how healthy they are. I'm just afraid I will get the taste back for chocolate. I feel great, especially my arthritic thumb.

Sugar causes chronic inflammation. If you can decrease your sugar intake, you'll also decrease inflammation in your body. Chronic and excessive inflammation causes not only pain, but also diseases like heart disease, diabetes, obesity, dementia, Alzheimer's, cancer, and allergies. Read labels! When I purchase my healthy protein bars, I make sure I don't buy anything that has more than 5-10 grams of sugar per serving. According to the American Heart Association (AHA), the maximum amount of added sugars you should eat in a day are:

- Men: 150 calories per day (37.5 grams or 9 teaspoons)
- Women: 100 calories per day (25 grams or 6 teaspoons)

Added sugar is found mostly in processed foods and drinks. Other common forms of sugar are honey, maple syrup, coconut sugar, turbinado sugar, high fructose corn syrup, corn syrup, sucrose, fructose, glucose, and dextrose. Some may be perceived as healthier choices. Don't be fooled. Your body sure isn't. Too much sugar is too much, no matter the source. Reduce your sugar intake by limiting soft drinks, fruit juice, candy, and baked goods.

There are other pro-inflammatory foods besides added sugar and they include processed foods, unhealthy fats (including saturated and trans-fats), preservatives, and refined carbohydrates. According to Mayo Clinic Family Physician Dr. Ardon, deep-fried foods, pastries, processed cereals, white rice, white potatoes, breads, and red meat are also pro-inflammatory foods.

Doesn't it sound and feel better to eat foods that fight inflammation? Like detoxing your system - nice and clean! Not only does it sound good, it IS good for your body and brain, plus you will FEEL much better and be motivated to be stronger. All the pieces work together. Stronger... Happier.... Better life... Quality of life.... Longevity!

Here are some guidelines from the Mayo Clinic for anti-inflammatory eating:

- **Whole plant foods** have the anti-inflammatory nutrients that your body needs. Examples: fruits, veggies, whole grains, and legumes.
- **Antioxidants** help prevent, delay, or repair some types of cell and tissue damage. Examples: colorful fruits and veggies like berries, leafy greens, beets, and avocados, as well as beans and lentils, whole grains, ginger, turmeric, and green tea.
- **Omega-3** fatty acids play a role in regulating your body's inflammatory process and could help regulate pain related to inflammation. Examples of healthy fats: fish like salmon, tuna, herring, and mackerel, as well as smaller amounts in walnuts, pecans, ground flaxseed, and soy.
- **Decrease red meat.**
- **Cut processed foods.**

Eating for Optimal Brain Function

Meaningful and life changing experiences, like decreasing inflammation and pain, can motivate change in our eating habits for life. The bonus may be weight loss and getting in better shape. However, if weight loss is the sole goal, and you have tried for years and it hasn't worked, you have to dig deeper to find other reasons to eat healthier. I've seen people lose weight when they are happier with their lives. I've seen people lose weight when they've discovered a new passion in life that requires them to be in shape. I've seen my own weight loss when I got motivated about **eating for the health of my brain** since both my parents had dementia. It was not my intention to lose weight - my sole motivation was to get my brain as healthy as possible. Sorry to say, this is something you can't see the positive results from right away - dementia will either show up or not as we age. That's why the science behind having a healthy brain is even more important to me than things that I can see and feel, like my strong and pain-free body.

I came across the book *Genius Foods* by coincidence and it changed my life. In the introduction of the book, I related immediately with the author Max Lugavere, who wrote the book while researching solutions for his mother's Alzheimer disease. Max writes *"This book is a guide to attaining optimal brain function with the pleasant effect of minimizing dementia risk - all according to the latest science."* The book had such an impact on me that I made it part of a topic of one of my Holistic Fitness Retreats "Boost Your Brain Health & Fitness." One of his suggestions was to take extra care of the health of the brain by intermittent fasting. As with anything, before recommending my clients to try it, I test it first on myself. The words *intermittent fasting* took me back to my high school days of exploring fasting, which I absolutely hated. It just made me think about food all the time. Based on that experience 40 years ago, I truly doubted that I would last more than a day. To my great surprise, intermittent fasting is quite different from pure fasting. I have been doing it for a year every day and now it is part of my life - I love it. It keeps my brain healthy (fingers crossed) and as a bonus it keeps my body weight regular. I've dropped down to my high school weight and kept it for a whole year without too much of an effort. Not that I was ever overweight before, but I do confess to the fact that I've struggled in the past with weight gain of five and sometimes ten pounds at times.

Intermittent Fasting for a Healthier Brain

What is intermittent fasting? It means giving the brain a break from food for 12-16 hours a day. This is not a new concept; in fact fasting has been utilized for health and longevity for centuries.

How does intermittent fasting work? There are different ways to do it. The most common one is the 16:8 ratio, meaning 16 hours of fasting and 8 hours of eating. According to the Genius Foods book, women's hormone systems may be more sensitive to warning signs of food shortage and should start with 12-14 hrs. Note that prolonged fasts may adversely affect fertility. As with anything, consult your doctor prior to trying it. One of my elderly clients was advised against intermittent fasting by her doctor.

During the eating period, make sure you feed your brain and body with healthy fuels - healthy fats, proteins, and fibrous vegetables. Starving is not an option. It is life threatening to not provide your body with enough nutrition to operate and function optimally. In addition, it triggers starvation mode, which means the body will fight to hang on to all energy (calories) from all sources (fat, protein, and carbohydrates). It will not let go of any calories. This is what happens when people lack knowledge on how to eat to lose weight. They think, "I'll just stop eating." Dangerous decision! Food is fuel! If you don't have fuel in the tank of your car, it won't drive. Same applies to the body - if you don't eat, the body won't function.

During the fasting period, drink as much water as you wish. You can also drink tea and coffee, but do not add anything like milk or cream. That defeats the purpose of letting the body take a break from digesting the food. Choose what window of fasting that works for you. Some skip breakfast and start the first food intake at 11am and the last at 7pm. Some skip dinner and start eating at 7am and finish eating at 3pm. It's a very personal choice. Make it work for YOU!

Why would you do intermittent fasting? We adapted to the brains of our preagricultural ancestors, who were without food for long periods of time due to an irregular food supply. In today's society (or most modern societies), we are overfeeding from the moment we wake up to the moment we go to bed and we miss out on the amazing benefits from taking a break from eating for 12-16 hrs.

Some of the Amazing Benefits from Intermittent Fasting

1. Reduces inflammation by helping the body to cleanse itself; for example: to get rid of old or damaged cells.

2. Enhances fat loss by burning fat as fuel instead of sugar because all the sugar stores have been used up during fasting.

3. Improves insulin sensitivity because the body is taking a long enough break from digesting food to lower the insulin levels, allowing the body to re-sensitize to insulin again.

4. Stimulates the production of new brain cells and nerve tissue (neurogenesis), which is linked to increased brain performance, memory, mood, and focus.

5. Promotes neuroplasticity, which is the brain's lifelong capacity to change and rewire itself in response to the stimulation of new learning, creating new connections between the neurons, and adapting to new circumstances.

6. Naturally boosts human growth hormone (HGH) to provide healthy anti-aging, repair, neuroprotective (preserving brain health and performance), and longevity benefits in addition to helping preserve lean tissue (muscles).

7. Increases the creation of mitochondria, the batteries for your cells, taking the food you eat and turning it into ENERGY.

As you can see a lot of the benefits of intermittent fasting is for our brains. Yay! Many motivational answers to my big "why" I only eat from 11am-7pm every day. Am I super strict? No, there are some days I eat earlier and some evenings I eat later, but all in all I'm doing it 95% of the time. I make it work for me. Again, my main motivation is to take care of my brain.

What is YOUR strong "why" that will motivate you to make healthier food choices consistently? Dig deep to find reasons. Think about the whole picture and all the benefits from living a healthy active lifestyle, including eating healthy, exercising, and practicing mindfulness. Ask yourself quality questions to find the answer. Be brave. Sit long enough with one question until you have found a truthful answer from deep within.

- What worries me most about the future?
- Am I holding on to something I need to let go of?
- What matters most in my life?
- Why do I matter?
- If not now, then when?

The only weight loss information I will give you is to educate yourself so you'll have realistic expectations in case losing weight is your goal. Keeping your body weight in control is due to 80% of what you eat and 20% of how you exercise. As a matter of fact, you should know that one pound of your body weight contains 3,500 calories. If you would like to lose one pound a week, which is a recommended approach to keep the weight off for good, then you have to create a deficit of 500 calories per day. Combine decreasing your food intake and increasing your exercising. It's so much easier to consume calories than to get rid of them. Think about my 300 calorie Starbucks chocolate chip cookie. Get rid of that one! Then add a **brisk** 30-minute walk that burns up to 200 calories, and voila! There's your daily deficit.

Note that your speed and your body weight will determine your caloric expenditure. Walking burns anywhere from 90 to 200 calories in 30 minutes. You burn fewer calories if you walk at the strolling rate of a 30-minute mile. You burn more calories walking at the brisk rate of a 17-minute mile. The more you weigh and the less fit you are, the more calories are burned walking for 30 minutes. If walking hurts your joints, then do Nordic Walking, which also burns more calories than regular walking.

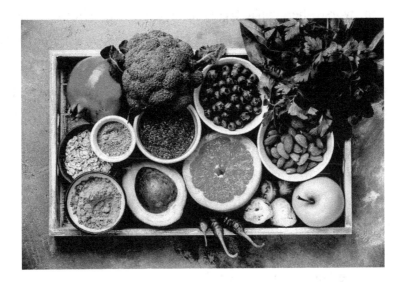

Changing Eating Habits

Now that you have explored what motivates you to make life changes, it's time to provide practical ways to improve your eating habits.

1. **Replace one unhealthy eating habit with a new healthy one**

   Drastic changes usually don't last for more than two weeks. Make one small adjustment at a time and you will be ok for a lifetime. One way to alter your eating habits is to replace an old bad eating habit with a new good one. Think it through, be realistic, and write it down. It is very powerful.

   For example, put your snacks on a plate instead of eating them from the package to help control how much you eat. Change a bad snack to a healthy snack like nuts, but still be disciplined with the portion by placing them in a small bowl.

2. **Change your kitchen into a healthy environment**

   We keep our food in the kitchen and sometimes we eat in the kitchen. Change that environment to an inviting and healthy place. Put inspirational quotes up on the fridge to set your mind up for success. Place your workout calendar for the month on the fridge to stay motivated. Put up photos of you looking and feeling healthy as an inspiration. Do a cleanup of all unwanted food. Having temptations lying around is the worst when you're trying to eat better. Only buy one cookie instead of a whole package. Don't deprive yourself, but don't set up any traps either! If you say you need to have snacks for the kids and grandkids, I say sure, but make them healthy snacks. Imagine how they will grow up eating healthy and making it part of their lifestyle. You've given them the best investment there is - their health!

3. **Surround yourself with supportive and like-minded people**

   Making changes is hard enough. Having somebody constantly tempting you with food that you're trying your hardest to stay away from can be torture. Be around people who will support you. If you don't eat sugar anymore and somebody offers a cake at their birthday party just say, "No, thank you." No need for any deeper explanations, because then you will have everyone saying, "Oh c'mon it's my birthday, just one piece of cake." Well, one piece may be all it will take to get you back to your old bad habits. It's like offering a cigarette to a smoker who quit smoking a week ago. Would you offer them a cigarette and say, "Oh, c'mon it's just one cigarette - c'mon keep me company." Sugar is just as addictive as nicotine. We crave it, but when we don't have it for a while, we crave it less and eventually we don't crave it at all. Wouldn't that be heaven? To not crave sweets? If I could get rid of my Swedish sweet tooth, you can too. Give it a try. Be strong and get support from people who want you to succeed. What do you have to lose? Nothing! You'll only gain benefits like having more energy. So worth it!

4. **Don't obsess about missing out on an old unhealthy eating habit**

Changing eating habits doesn't equal deprivation. Make small changes and have healthy substitutes instead. The more you think about your old eating habit, the harder it will be. Instead, focus on the benefits you experience when you replace the old bad eating habit with a new good one. Pat yourself on the back and confirm that you are proud of yourself for making these healthy changes.

5. **Preparation is key**

If you come home starving and there is nothing to eat that is healthy and fast to make, you will fail. You will grab the thing that will satisfy your hunger. That's why you need to prepare. This is not about just saying, "I'm going to eat healthier." This is about taking serious action to clean up your kitchen, to buy healthy snacks on the go, and to nourish a strong mind to say "no" when you're tempted by yourself or non-supportive people. Prepare the prior evening and decide what you will eat the next day, when you will move and exercise. If you buy groceries once a week, then make a plan for the week. The bottom line is that you need to have easy access to healthy food when you're hungry.

6. **Make a list of ten things you would change about your eating.**

Organize them so the easiest one ends up at the top of the list. We are going to cross off only one at a time. Crossing off an item on a to-do list is a wonderful feeling of accomplishment. Setting yourself up for success by taking action on the first and the easiest one is a smart move. One step at a time and very soon you will have crossed off your whole list. That's when you will see the most change in yourself, but like any journey, it starts with one step. Depending on how difficult one item is, I would take 2-3 weeks before I dive into trying out the next one on the list. Give it time. Really let it sink in and stick with you before moving on. We're talking about making changes for a lifetime and not just two weeks. Here are twelve examples to get you started:

1. Get rid of unhealthy food from the kitchen.
2. Eat something healthy at home prior to going to a party with tons of temptations. Feeling full will help limit the temptation to grab something unhealthy at the party.
3. Think before you eat. Be conscious of what you eat. Avoid eating randomly. Think before you eat something you will regret.
4. Plan all your meals and snacks for the following week.
5. Avoid shopping on an empty stomach.
6. Make it a habit to always read food labels.
7. Choose water instead of sodas and juices.
8. Avoid snacking before bedtime. Eating no later than three hours before bedtime will help you sleep better.
9. Eat slowly (place utensils down in between each bite) and chew well.
10. Make sure it is not dressing with salad but salad with some dressing.
11. Always sit down to eat. Avoid rushing and eating on the go. Enjoy every bite.
12. You don't have to say "yes" to any food or desserts offered to you to be polite. If they know you are watching what you eat, they are the rude ones for not respecting your decision.

How good of shape you're in depends 80% on what you eat and 20% on how you exercise. The goal with this chapter was to educate you on what it really takes to eat healthy and how that can maximize your brain capacity for a longer, happier life. Having a strong motivation for eating healthy will get you there not only faster, but you will be able to keep staying healthy for a lifetime. Focusing on weight loss is not what I recommend. Instead get motivated and pumped up from all the incredible benefits to have an optimal functioning brain. Wake up that brain of yours! Let's go to the next chapter to figure out how you can keep up the great work by selecting a 3-point support system, including YOU!

CHECK-IN #10: FEED YOUR BODY AND BRAIN

Now you have the information on what it means to eat healthy. Create your list of five things (or more) that you specifically need to change in regard to your eating habits. Start with the easier ones at the top. When you feel it is part of your life after about 2-3 weeks, cross it off. Time to take action on the next item on your list. Repeat until every item is crossed off from your list. Be patient. Celebrate each time you cross an item off!

My Personal Changing Eating Habit List:

1. _____

2. _____

3. _____

4. _____

5. _____

_____

_____

_____

_____

_____

_____

_____

"Go confidently in the direction of your dreams.
Live the life you have imagined."
~Henry David Thoreau

CHAPTER 11:

Your Success Team

How are you doing? Excited and empowered? Wonderful! Not to take that euphoric feeling away from you, but let's prepare for potential obstacles popping up along the way. It's better to deal with them now when you're feeling great, rather than when you may be feeling down. I am asking you to make a commitment to incorporate a new healthy lifestyle. Resistance will come up. Believe me, when you get over the hump, and make these practices part of your daily routine, your life is going to be amazing. The question is how to sustain this lifestyle for more than two weeks. The answer is to build, nourish, and maintain a support system around you so you can change for a lifetime.

Three Ways to Successfully Stick to the Long-Term Plan

If you are lacking a success team, when obstacles come up, they may prevent you from reaching your long-term goals. It's easy to do something for a couple of weeks, but to keep that healthy lifestyle up, believe me, you will need solid and reliable support. In this chapter I will help you select your Success Team which consists of you, your closest family & friends, and your health & medical team.

Let's start with how you can support yourself.

YOU Supporting YOU:

If not now, then when? You are the only person standing in your way. Let the past be the past. Today is a new day. Make the future count. Your health is a huge investment for your future. Make the changes in your life that you want, not what somebody else wants. Live your life. Be responsible for your actions. Make good choices from now on. Be your own cheerleader for your success and change those negative voices into productive and positive ones. Remember your "why" that will motivate you to make healthier choices consistently.

This is a long-term plan and you have to be ready. This is driven by you and nobody else. That's why the strength training workout in this book has no equipment - to make it easier for you to get started right away, from anywhere. Zero excuses. The same goes for the cardio segment - you can walk anytime and anywhere. Further down the road, you will need some basic fitness equipment for other workouts. You may also want some poles to go Nordic Walking to burn more calories than regular walking, and to take the weight off the joints while strengthening the upper body.

So, what are you waiting for? Let's get you ready! Where will the place be located where you meditate, work out, and eat? Setting up your life to be supported like this at a bigger level needs some preparation.

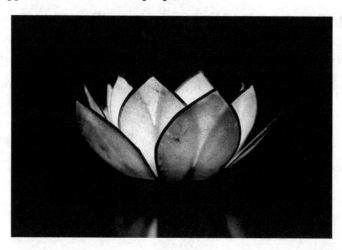

First, locate a sacred space for practicing mindfulness and meditation to set up your mindset for success. Is there a sacred space in your home? Find a place where you can easily sit down to spend 20 minutes by yourself, undisturbed and uninterrupted. You may have to negotiate with your family unless you live by yourself. Then you only need to decide where. How can you make it a special and sacred space? An easy way to increase the ambiance is to light a candle. Create this space and make it very special.

Your movement space is for physical movement, including trigger release, warm-up, dynamic drills, strength training workouts, cardio workouts, and static stretching. Will you do it indoors at home or at a gym? Or outdoors? Except for walking, Nordic Walking and some Dynamic Drills, which can be done outdoors, all you need is a space for a yoga mat to fit, plus some additional space around the mat. If you have a hard surface like wood or cement, the yoga mat needs to be a thicker exercise mat so it's comfortable to lie on.

Your meal space is usually the kitchen, but it includes any areas where you consume your healthy foods and drinks (water!). Only you know what those specific areas are. My recommendation is that you make sure those areas are filled with healthy choices - especially if you were to get into a "hangry" (hungry + angry) state of mind and are ready to grab anything edible around you.

Planning will definitely set you up for success. Decide on a day that is dedicated to planning your **meals and drinks** for the week. That way you can be ready to follow the shopping list when you go grocery shopping without getting sidetracked by temptations. Knowing you have everything healthy at hand will keep your mind from racing when those hunger feelings show up without any warning signs. You may be so involved in a project and then BANG! you realize you're starving. That's when it's extra smart to have healthy choices in stock for an easy grab.

Decide the days you are going to **work ou**t for the week. It is easier to plan and keep the workouts if you schedule the same days every week. For example, on Mondays, Thursdays, and Saturdays I do my strength training workouts. On

Tuesdays, Fridays, and Sundays I do my cardio training workouts. Wednesday is my active resting day - no workouts. Make sure you also have appropriate workout clothes and shoes to be comfortable. Regardless what time you exercise during the day, always prepare your workout clothes the day before. One fewer excuse to use. "Oh, I can't find my favorite workout shoes" and then you end up running around 20 minutes searching for them when you could have - you guessed it - worked out already for 20 minutes. Enter these days into your calendar where you keep all other meetings, appointments, and dates. Color code the schedule if possible. Make the commitment to your workout days and times sacred. If you are not healthy, you can't take care of anyone else. Just saying. You have to be the priority.

Tracking is another great way to make sure you stay on track with a healthy new lifestyle. Setting goals has to be measurable. You can't just guesstimate. Know how many steps you take daily by wearing a pedometer either attached to your waistline or a watch-like pedometer you wear on your wrist.

Tracking your workouts can easily be done by just printing a 30-day calendar, filling out the days you do strength and the days you do cardio, and marking it off each time you finish. Place it on the fridge so you can see the progress with your own eyes. Members of the *Monthly and Annual Memberships Online* receive a new 30-day calendar every month designed exactly for this purpose.

Keeping track of what you eat can be loaded with tons of resistance. If you write it down, you have to acknowledge you consumed it. There's no way around it. Be truthful with yourself even if it means looking at lots of food you should not eat on that sheet of paper. You have to start somewhere and a new relationship with you lasts longer and is more successful if you're being honest with yourself from the start. As you learn and change to better eating habits, it will feel good to look at all the healthy choices you are writing down compared to when you started. A few more things to track can be your medical readings like blood pressure, cholesterol, resting heart rate, etc. If you're really brave, you may also want to see what the scale says, or better yet, how your favorite pair of jeans or dress fits or doesn't fit now but how it changes for the better each week you try them on.

Even with you being fully prepared, the unknown and the uncertainty still may throw you off track. How can you prevent this incredible plan of yours from going out the window? Here are a few scenarios that I have seen with clients and customers that work with me either one-one-one or as a group at my classes, workshops and retreats. Anything that can get in your way - here are some solutions on how to handle it.

Getting Sick

Getting sick is your body's way of saying you have to stop and rest. Sleeping is the best medicine to fast recovery. Sleep, eat healthy, drink water is what I do when I get sick - which is very rare. Hopefully, you have the kitchen stocked with healthy foods and snacks. If not, please ask somebody to go grocery shopping for you or just order meals from a healthy local restaurant. When you're not sleeping all the time anymore, you may want to start with some gentle movements in bed by just moving the joints. Lying down a lot can make you really stiff. When you are able to get up and move around a little bit, try the foam roller and some easy trigger release places like the buttocks. When you are ready to exercise, start with some easy strength training exercises if you've had some upper respiratory challenges. For your cardio, just go for some short and slow-paced walks. When your upper respiratory situation is fully recovered, start doing some easy cardio, gently challenging your body by walking at a faster pace for a longer duration. Watch out for residuals. If you push your body too soon and too hard, you may end up back in that bed again. Be wise and listen to your body even though you're sick and tired of resting. Most importantly, follow the directions from your physician. Never start working out where you left off before you got sick. Gradually build your body back up over a few weeks. Working out on a regular basis will make it easier for you to bounce back to where you were in just a couple of weeks. Be patient.

Keep practicing mindfulness so your strong mindset can support your body. Your body will feel so much better if you keep those positive affirmations up. A client and friend of mine survived cancer a few years ago and I believe her strong commitment to affirmations helped her through it. She is one of the most positive and most grateful people I know. Let her be your inspiration. Practice those affirmations whether you're on top of the world or at your lowest point. Mind-Body connection!

Getting Injured

An injury can put an end to working out if it involves the whole body. If only a small part of your body is injured, like a hand, you can still go for walks. If only your foot is injured, you can still do some upper body strength training exercises, including the core. Again, the main thing is that you follow the doctor's and/or the physical therapist's orders. The same advice applies as if you were sick: return gradually and gently to avoid any re-injuries. Just because you have an injury doesn't mean that you stop practicing mindfulness and eating healthy. Even though you feel down and frustrated, don't let one injury hold you back from making progress. This is where a strong mindset and support from your family and friends really matter. If your whole team of support is on the same page as you are, they will keep supporting your new healthy way of living. The injury sucks, but it is just a temporary set-back. Don't let that throw off everything that you have worked so hard to build. Stay strong within your body and mind!

Experiencing Pain

Feeling pain can be really scary if you are not used to that feeling. Have you ever gotten a really bad charley horse cramp in your calf or inner thigh? Everything around you suddenly seem to come to a halt as you desperately try to activate the opposite muscle to trick the cramping muscles to relax. Pain can be so bad that it takes your breath away. If you experience pain that is more excruciating than a cramp, you obviously go to the ER. If the pain is less, but persistent, you want to make an appointment with your doctor to get a diagnosis to figure out what to do. If the pain is so little that you don't need to see a doctor, plus the pain disappears after a week, you can most likely return to working out, but be aware of why the pain appeared. Is it your weak link in your body? Was it the lower back pain? Do you need to focus on building a stronger core? Having a good and well-educated trainer helping you get you stronger is a wise investment. If the pain is an ongoing vicious cycle, you definitely want a doctor's opinion and maybe start physical therapy. After the PT sessions run out, I highly recommend you get your trainer involved so the person can communicate with the PT so there is a flow in the transition from PT to working out with the trainer. Whatever you decide to do, keep up everything else that is helping you live a healthier lifestyle.

New Work Assignments

What happens if your boss gives you a big new assignment that will increase your workload and hours? Adjust your schedule. The busier you get, the more important it is to prioritize your health. The assignment is probably a temporary change in your life. Don't let it interrupt your healthy way of living. Time is more precious than before. More than ever you have to schedule everything - both work and workouts. Take advantage of every minute in the day. I'd suggest you schedule the workouts first thing in the morning, so you only need to focus on physical movement like going for walks to prevent the body from getting stiff for the rest of the day. Sprinkling in some walks during the day will also give your mind a mental break from the intense work assignment. That will make you even more productive. Adding your positive affirmations on your walks will further enhance the work productivity and creativity. With that intense pace it is even more important that you keep a healthy lifestyle, especially getting enough sleep. Enough sleep will keep your brain more focused and alert and provide clarity to any project, maximizing the success of the assignment from your boss.

Travel for Business or Pleasure

Depending on the length of the trip, you will either experience small or large interruptions. If it's a week, you'll still be able to get back to where you were when you left off. If it's longer than a week, you have to put more energy and effort to make the new healthy lifestyle work for you while traveling. Practicing mindfulness is something you can do anywhere and anytime. Doing strength training workouts can be done in a hotel room and you can use the nine exercises from this book since no equipment is required. The cardio workouts may be tricky unless you have access to a gym or if you can safely walk outdoors where you're staying. The good news is that we all know how to do video conferencing from the Coronavirus Pandemic in 2020. Your trainer can keep working you out even if you travel. The only challenge is the time zone and making your schedules work. Eating healthy may be the toughest one, but again, if you plan and prepare, you can make that work too. Unless you travel internationally, go to a grocery store you are familiar with to get your healthy (prepared) meals and snacks. It may not be ideal, but today with food delivery and all, you should be able to eat healthy while traveling, at least for 80% of your trip. If you do your best, you will be happy with yourself. In the end, that's what counts!

Let's continue with how you can get support from people around you.

Your Team Supporting YOU:

The most important support system besides yourself are all the people you are around. Who do you spend most time with? Whose advice do you most value? Write down your top three people. Make them your inner circle allies. Make sure they understand what you are doing and how incredibly important it is to you to adopt a healthy lifestyle for life. They need to support you and not tempt you, and help to minimize any temptations at dinner parties or any social gatherings serving foods and drinks.

When I arrived in Los Angeles in 1989, I faced three tough years before I received my green card. I had to return to Sweden quite often. During one of those trips, I asked my parents to keep supporting my decision even though it seemed too much work to be able to stay and work legally in the USA. They have always supported me no matter what I have done with my life. Well, except for one time when my dad sat me down and asked, "Why can't you travel when you have graduated University?" I said, "Because then I may not feel like it. It is now that my heart tells me to explore the world by traveling." He was not happy, but he understood how important it was for me to follow my heart. When I graduated with a master's degree in PE from the Swedish Sports University in 1988, he was very happy. I think because I was child number six and I had always done things my way, they knew it was important for me to have their support. Even though they wanted their baby to stay home in Sweden, they still supported my decision. That's love! Make sure your team has your back too. They really have to understand to what degree this is important to you. If they love you enough, they will support your decision and help you.

Maybe they will even climb onboard. I have a client who comes to every single one of my classes, workshops, and retreats. She made a commitment to herself to get healthy at age 60. In addition to all my events, she entered a walking challenge almost a year in advance - it involved walking over a bridge with quite a steep incline. She conquered that bridge and I was so proud of her! Now she has turned her husband and sister on to a healthy lifestyle as well. That's her family and she wants them to get and stay healthy too. By the way, her daughter joined her for the walking race. Isn't that fantastic? She has involved the whole family into the process of leading a healthy lifestyle. Makes it easier to achieve and to keep!

If you don't have any family members locally, then maybe you have a friend that can be your walking partner and workout buddy. To have somebody you have to be accountable to and show up for takes away any excuses. One time I trained for a half marathon in Sweden during the wintertime. If I hadn't made an agreement to meet my friend every morning at 6am, I would not have trained for it. Summertime, yes, but in the wintertime with the snow and the even colder wind factor. No way! See what friends and some support can do? It works wonders

Let's finish with how you can get even more support from your health and medical team

Your Health and Medical Team Supporting YOU:

Part of your health and medical team can be doctors, chiropractors, physical therapists, massage therapists, personal fitness trainers, etc. Make sure you build your health, fitness, and medical team by asking friends and family for referrals. It is important to have a medical care team that is on the same page, and speaks the same language, so you don't get conflicting information. (Unless, of course, you need a second opinion with a complicated diagnosis.)

Deal with egos as little as possible. Everyone should have your best interests at heart and not their own. If something is outside my expertise, I have absolutely no problem with referring my clients to other professionals on the health, fitness, and medical referral team. Here is where your support system is even beyond me. I know some of the best people to serve you. My support continues outside of me and we work as a team. That way you can smoothly transition from working with a physical therapist back to me as your personal fitness trainer. I integrate the physical therapist's prescribed exercises and guidelines into the workouts. You may first want to stay with the Nordic Body Reboot Program for a few weeks. When you're ready to return 100%, you return not to where you left off, but to where it is wise for your body to restart.

My method works and is a unique approach for the 50+ age group. Now is not the time to jam your joints into crazy positions, jump as high as you can, or run as fast as you can. This is the time to build up slowly with tons of awareness and respect for your body to prevent injuries while you're getting and staying strong. Age with great confidence. Make that body last as long as possible before you start replacing body parts and/or have surgeries. Modern medicine is quite amazing, but surgery should be a last option as it can add a whole new set of complications.

I personally train and coach people from my heart and with compassion without shaming them for what their bodies can't do. I gently have them step up and build up to feel safe and trust me. I'm big on honoring your body. We know we are going to live much longer. You need to ask yourself, "How can I best take care of my body?" Well, you've come to the right place, I specialize in giving instructions on how to take care of your body and mind after 50. Yes, it takes a lot of patience and awareness, but if you take your time to do it little by little, you'll realize this approach is much different from jumping as high as you can or running as fast as you can to burn as many calories as you can.

I don't believe in extremes. If something doesn't feel good, try fixing it and then keep going. Don't stop moving your body or feeding your brain with negativity like, "I'm old, I can't do this anymore." There is a middle road. You don't have to think, "I'm going to push myself through this pain" and run marathons and end up going in for surgery after surgery to fix you so you can keep thrashing your body. Nor should you totally stop moving if there's pain in your body. The bottom line is that you have to stop and connect with your body - do a body scan - and accept where you are right now. Honor and respect the body. Make a plan with help and advice from your medical care team including your fitness trainer and move forward from there.

Are you afraid of something breaking in your body and then you have to suffer in your 80's and 90's? This system will help you to stay consistently in shape and consistently feed your mind and brain with premium thoughts and fuel - so you don't have to be afraid you will break anything. This system is created to prevent injuries. What crazy stuff you may do outside the workouts is on you, but this system is designed to gradually build you up to keep you strong and confident as you age into your 60's, 70's, 80's, 90's, 100's, and beyond. My clients are not only my inspiration, but they have given me the wisdom and the knowledge for me to be able to say today, "I know what does and doesn't work to age successfully." It's been 28 years of working out the 50+ crowd - I have seen it all – the good and the bad. If you're in your 40's, this is a goldmine for you to ensure you invest correctly into your health and future. Many of my clients say, "I wish I had started with this earlier in life." You don't have to be past 50 to get the benefits from this book. You can be a teenager and benefit from this!

Just a few years ago, I gave my niece and her boyfriend a private workout with me as a high school graduation gift. I had to correct their techniques and I saw they were heading down the injury road. They got an early headstart. My niece had joined the cross country and track and field teams. There were plenty of horror stories of how they trained and pushed through injuries. It is frightening and so irresponsible of the coaches. So yes, teenagers will benefit from reading this book as well. It is just based on my experience with the 50+ crowd since 1992. Any age can use this book as a base, and then build from there to any crazy or intense activity you want.

The last piece of the puzzle is almost the most important one – brain health. Through meditation/mindfulness, exercising, and eating well, you also take good care of your brain, but if you want to invest into the best functioning and most powerful brain, there's more you can do. You need to prioritize keeping your brain healthy on a daily basis by eating healthy, exercising, getting enough sleep, minimizing stress, socializing, and learning something new.

The brain is an amazing computer that we need to keep healthy throughout life. Some of it we can control with exercise, eating well, thinking well, and trying new things to keep stimulating the brain. Unfortunately, some of it we can't control. We don't know if we'll end up with dementia diseases or muscle atrophy diseases, etc. Regardless, stay strong in both body and mind. If something out of your control were to happen to you, it's always better to face it with feeling as strong as possible (physically and mentally).

From the headquarters (your brain), everything can make the rest of the body work. The brain sends signals to the heart to pump blood. The brain sends signals to the muscles to contract and release. The brain is like a conductor and if she (the conductor) has received premium fuel (nutrition), oxygen from the blood (exercise), is relaxed and stress free, is surrounded by supportive friends & family, gets enough sleep every night, and tries to learn new things in life, she can successfully conduct a beautiful orchestra with everything in the body cooperating optimally. Would you like your brain to operate like this too? Today it's possible!

It was previously believed that the brain just kept on losing brain cells as we age, but today there are many studies showing that we can make changes in the brain (brain plasticity). For example, meditation has proved to help change the plasticity of the brain.

I have created a simple checklist below for your Success Team to take everything into account!

6 Ways to Take Care of That Beautiful Brain of Yours

1. **Nutrition** - what you eat directly affects the structure and function of your brain and, ultimately, your mood.

2. **Exercise** - increases the blood flow to deliver oxygen and nutrients for the brain to operate optimally. Improves mood, sleep, and reduces stress and anxiety. Problems in these areas frequently cause or contribute to cognitive impairment.

3. **Sleep** - helps restore the brain by flushing out toxins that build up during waking hours.

4. **De-Stress** - stress decreases amounts of klotho, a hormone that keeps toxins in the brain, in check. The hippocampus (structure of the brain) regulates motivation, emotion, learning, and memory, and protects you from aging. Chronic stress (cortisol spikes) can lead to memory impairments.

5. **Socializing** - provides sources of support, reduces stress, combats depression, and enhances intellectual stimulation. Happy, long-term relationships and having a purpose in life have shown significant protective effects against age-related cognitive impairment.

6. **Stimulating Intellectual Activities** - on a regular basis, significantly lowers the risk of dementia. Learn a new language, take a class, or read the newspaper is some advice from Dr. Small, director of UCLA Longevity Center.

You can have everything your heart desires. Start challenging yourself! Try new things, get out of your comfort zone, drive a different route, learn a new skill, and never ever say you can't do it. Because we know that if the brain can change, so can YOU!

Share the system in this book with your Success Team so they can better support you. You will succeed when you follow the system in this book with guidelines on what to do and how much. In the appendix of this book, you can find exactly how to structure your strength training workouts and your walking/Nordic Walking workouts. In addition to this book, I can offer you support either via live or online events. If you live close to Los Angeles, you can come to my local live events like Nordic Walking classes, Strong Body + Mind Workshops, or Holistic Fitness Retreats. Every event has an amazing topic related to aging successfully. If you're interested in hosting one of my events for your group of ten or more closer to where you live, please email us at info@nordicbody.com. I can create a group for any location, indoors or out! No matter where you live, you can always get my support online. I offer different packages of *Monthly or Annual Memberships Online*. Go to https://nordicbody.com/wakeup to find out about your free trial offer.

CHECK-IN #11: YOUR SUCCESS TEAM

Start selecting your Success Team. Put a name in one of the three groups. Write how that person can support your healthy lifestyle. Your name will always appear in group one, so brainstorm how you can support yourself in different ways and situations.

1. You

_____

_____

_____

2. Friend/Family

_____

_____

_____

3. Health, Fitness and Medical team

_____

_____

_____

Betty Dasteel - 9TH DECADE

The first time I met Betty, I was taken by her sharp mind and sparkling blue eyes full of life and curiosity. She is 98 and still lives on her own with very little help. Isn't this what we all strive for in life? To be able to stay independent and live at home as long as possible! Most people her age are either dead or living in nursing homes. There are many wonderful active living communities for people 55+. For some, that solution is a blessing. To be around other people to fight the main issues we fear as we age - isolation, loneliness, and depression. Their batteries get recharged and they get a second chance to live a more meaningful life. Betty never had to worry about that. She has an innate zest for life. Betty has lived an interesting long life, traveling to many countries, and even living in a few due to her husband's Naval Officer position. They met on a successful blind date in Los Angeles and had many happy years of marriage with three sons. Before she became a homemaker, she went to Stanford University to study Biology and Physical Therapy, so she definitely understands the importance of taking care of her body. Even during the coronavirus, she insisted on working out with me at her home. We both dressed in masks, gloves, and gowns, plus keeping six feet apart. Once, many years ago, she took time off from working out because she was afraid the pain in her lower back would get worse. Now she knows it reduces the pain instead. She doesn't want to make that mistake again.

When I asked her, "Do you think our workouts benefit you?" she answered without hesitation, "I certainly do!" During the last four years of working out with me, she feels she has gotten stronger, can move more normally, and with more knowledge of what to do. However, every session she starts with saying, "Today I'm really bad. I don't think I can do much." Then she surprises both of us and finishes the whole program. At the end she says, "Oh I feel much better." We both chuckle and her blue eyes sparkle even brighter. During the four years, there have only been two times when she has not been able to complete the whole program. One was due to feeling overwhelmed and stressed. That's when I started to add meditation prior to us exercising. When I consulted with her doctors, they agreed it was a perfect idea to work on her breathing to manage her high blood pressure prior to working out. If her blood pressure is still too high, I modify the program to only do active stretching while sitting down. Fortunately, we haven't had to do this lately.

Betty deals with pain in her back due to arthritis and scoliosis. When the doctors look at the x-rays of her back, they think for sure that it is a person that is bound to a wheelchair. Betty does not even own a wheelchair. She uses a walker and a cane to get around. She knows that by moving more on a daily basis she feels better. I asked her, "What is the one thing you would like to share with everyone who is in their 50's and up?" "Keep moving the body," she says. So, folks, listen to Betty and keep moving that body of yours! She is 98 and she knows what she is talking about! She's been around the block.

~*Betty Dasteel, age 98, Los Angeles, CA*

"Life isn't about finding yourself.

Life is about creating yourself."

~George Bernard Shaw

CHAPTER 12:

Anything is Possible At Any Age

Now that you have a stronger body and mind, you can do anything. So, go out there in the world and go after what you've always dreamed. From our expansive time together, your body and mind are aligned to support you through anything you set your mind to. Get that bucket list out! Maybe you want to be even braver and reinvent yourself? Is your initial reaction, "No, Malin, I can't. I'm too old." Oh, really? What is too old for you? To me "old" is the day I am no longer curious about life. Until then, watch out! I have so much to do in this lifetime, I think I have to live to be 120. Would you like to join me?

I have a "zest for life" and if you are wondering why you feel better with a skip in your step, I have passed it on to you. "Zest for life" means an embodiment of enjoyment and enthusiasm for what surrounds you. Let's tap into THAT energy! To further pique your curiosity, ask these deep quality questions:

- What is your deepest desire?
- Where do you see yourself in one, five, or ten years?
- What is the dream you must accomplish to die happy and fulfilled?
- What stops you from fulfilling your dream?
- What do you want people to say about you at your funeral?

Keep exploring life till your last breath. Line up the inner desires with the outer. Take action. Adjust your thinking. Control your thoughts. Anything is now possible at any age. You felt like all this transformation would be a lot of work at the start of this book, and we did work hard, but ask yourself, "How is your life different now only a few short months later?" I bet you it feels better. To make a change takes work and effort, but soon this information will be second nature to you and an integral part of your life. Every thought starts in the mind and can result in a dream of yours coming true. The mind is powerful. Your body is powerful. You now have some tools to make changes in your life.

Open your heart to everything that is possible. Truly ask yourself, "What's next for me? What do I truly want to go after in life?" Tap into your true self! Sit down, close your eyes, and go deep inside to find the answer. If you are patient enough to sit quietly long enough, you will hear the answer from within you - from your inner wisdom. I believe we have all the answers within us. That has been my own journey during the last four years when I was reintroduced to spiritual meditation. Prior to that I only followed my heart, which served me very well. Now I also follow my inner wisdom, which feels like riding a wave. There is such a flow in life when you tap into that inner guidance.

My dreams make me feel alive. Manifesting desire is being awake to life. Be aware of every conscious moment, every breath, every thought. It's easy to get into a cycle of repetitive patterns that has shaped your life so far. Sometimes we go through life by just going through the motions to just get through the day. Then it starts all over the next day. Break that vicious cycle. Only you can do that. Think outside the box. Think of the bigger picture. Expand, thrive, and grow daily!

Bucket List

Let's start easy by gently asking what's on your bucket list? What are some things you would want to do before you leave planet Earth? Here are some examples.

1. Dance tango
2. Enter a 5k walk
3. Swim with wild dolphins
4. Travel to the Galápagos Islands
5. Skydiving

Your turn. Write at least five things on your bucket list.

1. _____

2. _____

3. _____

4. _____

5. _____

Reinvent Yourself

Let's dive deeper than the bucket list. Anytime someone I know thinks, "Has my ship sailed?" they turn around to see somebody their age or older doing that very feat! Makes you feel empowered that it CAN be done, right? Sprinkled throughout this book, you have read five stories from five people at five different decades reinventing themselves. The intention is to get you inspired to realize that YOU can do anything at any age. This is from somebody who had an age crisis at 22!

Elaine, age 56, was depressed from being an empty nester and could not find any motivation to get stronger and feeling better until she, by chance, found scuba diving. Charlene, age 61, experienced her soul being drained and decided to sell her company to follow her heart to the next chapter in her life to live a life with purpose. Bo failed to finish a challenging ski race at age 69 but set his mind and body to do it at age 70 and succeeded. Delphine, age 88, was not able to move for four years due to pain, but after six weeks of working out with me, she could walk a whole mile pain-free. Betty, age 98, kept working out with me despite back pain and she is living proof that you can get stronger and better at any age!

That's what happens if you push through. Elaine, Charlene, Bo, Delphine, and Betty set their minds to change regardless of their ages. That number didn't exist. Only the inner drive and the "why." I have had the privilege to watch

Delphine's journey up front and it's been an amazing transformation. That's why you need to have a big "why." Dive deeper. It will definitely motivate you to upgrade your life.

Map of Your Life

This eye-opening exercise will have you dividing your life into different decades and naming each decade with a theme that was the highlight of that decade. Doing this exercise could have single-handedly diverted me from age crisis because it felt so enriching and purposeful to see what I have done in my life in front of me in writing. More importantly, it's like looking at a map - how certain things have happened to take me to the next destination, job, experience, or adventure. Simultaneously, I look at that map and see where I want to go next. You can have the same experience with your life map. Status quo is very scary to me. I constantly want to move forward to explore life - you can definitely say that I have zest for life. This is your life - nobody else's.

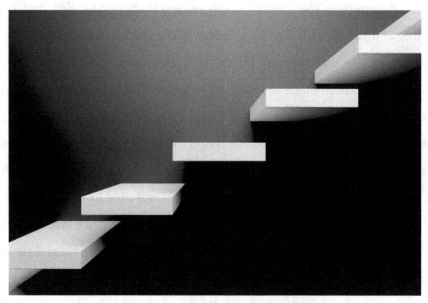

Let's explore what your next step may be

5 Action Steps to Find Your Next Step in Life

Let's walk down memory lane. Make sure you give yourself at least 15 minutes to get started with the "Map of Your Life" exercise. You can always return to do more. I'm sure memories will pop up when you least expect it. Grab the book and scribble them down.

1. On the next eleven empty pages, you will write **highlights and memories** (good or bad) from each decade up until your current decade. If a memory pops up, guesstimate what decade it took place and write it down on that page. For example, I was 14 when I was first kissed, and it was with 16-year-old Count Erik Stiernswärd! I will write that wonderful memory on the second decade (age 11-20).

2. Review all highlights/memories and mark each with a....

    a. **PLUS** symbol + after things that make you smile, make you feel proud or make your whole body feel warm of joy.

    b. **MINUS** symbol - after things that make you grit your teeth, make you feel regretful, or make the whole body shiver with a bad feeling.

3. Write down **dreams** you have had up until today. Try to place them within a decade you first think they appeared. Include the first thought about that dream.

4. Review all the dreams and mark:

    a. **DONE** after dreams you fulfilled even though they didn't turn out the way you expected. It's the fact that you went after your dreams that counts.

    b. **NOT DONE** after dreams you didn't pursue.

5. Finally, ask yourself what your desires and dreams are today? Choose one "not done" dream or a completely new emerging dream that you want to pursue right now.

DECADE #1: AGE 0-10

_____

_____

_____

_____

_____

_____

_____

_____

_____

_____

_____

_____

_____

_____

DECADE #2: AGE 11-20

_____

_____

_____

_____

_____

_____

_____

_____

_____

_____

_____

_____

_____

_____

_____

_____

_____

DECADE #3: AGE 21-30

_____

_____

_____

_____

_____

_____

_____

_____

_____

_____

_____

_____

_____

_____

_____

DECADE #4: AGE 31-40

_____

_____

_____

_____

_____

_____

_____

_____

_____

_____

_____

_____

_____

DECADE #5: AGE 41-50

DECADE #6: AGE 51-60

DECADE #7: AGE 61-70

DECADE #8: AGE 71-80

_____

_____

_____

_____

_____

_____

_____

_____

_____

_____

_____

_____

_____

_____

_____

DECADE #9: AGE 81-90

DECADE #10: AGE 91-100

_____

_____

_____

_____

_____

_____

_____

_____

_____

_____

_____

_____

_____

_____

_____

_____

DECADE #11: AGE 101-110+

If you see a pattern within one decade, you can name that decade. Give it a theme. The theme for my **DECADE #2: AGE 11-20** is "National Ranked Runner." The theme for my **DECADE #3: AGE 21-30** is "Travel & Master's Degree in Physical Education." That's why I'm always so excited about entering a new decade of my life because it means the start of a new chapter. There may be blank pages for your future decades. You get to fill in what those dreams and desires are. Perhaps some of those unrealized dreams will finally have their time in the sun!

The "Map of Your Life" exercise will show you how you have contributed to your life. You will see patterns in your purpose. We always want to feel needed and like we are contributing. Stay fulfilled till your last breath. Now you have the body and mind to accomplish anything, as well as the clarity.

What one dream did you write down in action step number five? Focus on that one dream and desire you want to pursue right now. There are many books written about how to pursue a dream. This is only an exercise to get you started, to get your feet wet, to build up your confidence to pursue it now that you have a strong body and mind to support you. The purpose of this book is to get you strong and keep you strong so you can live a fun, healthy and fulfilling life.

Besides health and fitness, another passion of mine is to set goals to make dreams come true with hard work, but also with inner wisdom manifestations. I'll leave you with three simple tips you can expand upon to make your dreams come true.

1. **Dream** - write your dreams down with as much specificity as possible.
2. **Plan** - make a plan on what needs to happen for the dreams to come true.
3. **Action** - enter action steps into your calendar to take daily action towards your dream.

Congratulations! You're on your way to pursue a dream with an awakened body and mind! You're tingling with excitement about your next step in life on a new level than ever before. How does that feel for your ultimate success? This is a lifestyle commitment and finding the motivation to continue is always the key. Use the mantras/positive affirmations presented in this book throughout the day. I'm a master at manifestation. I have a vision board with my dreams and desires in front of me in several places. Every morning starts out with me looking at those. Then I sit down to mediate. Set your day up the right way. Let's do this together! Let's go! Go live a life with passion and purpose no matter what your age is. Keep me updated and let me know how I can support you.

Having a big life with a happy healthy body and mind can be simpler than you think. At the end of the day, I believe these are the key ingredients you need to Wake Up Your Body and Mind to age successfully.

A CHECKLIST TO WAKE UP YOUR BODY + MIND AFTER 50+

- ☐ Practice mindfulness daily to reboot your mind and decrease stress.

- ☐ Roll away your aches and pains to reboot the body.

- ☐ Put your C.A.P. on to move correctly, fearlessly, and dynamically.

- ☐ Lead an active lifestyle, aiming for 10,000 steps daily to stay energized.

- ☐ Work out 30 minutes for 5-6 days a week to strengthen the bones, muscles, and heart.

- ☐ Take 1 active rest day/week to restore and to rebuild the body.

- ☐ Explore various ways of stretching to decrease stiffness and to stay flexible.

- ☐ Get a good night's sleep every night to cleanse the brain to stay more alert.

- ☐ Feed your brain and body with optimal fuel for best performance in life.

- ☐ Socialize with positive, like-minded, active people to keep your brain healthy.

- ☐ Get motivated from your support system to keep your healthy lifestyle for life.

- ☐ Live a life with passion and purpose at any age.

"From the bottom of my heart, I wish you to be your strongest in both your body and mind to live a fun, healthy, and fulfilling life!"

~ **Malin Svensson**

APPENDIX A

The Nordic Body System and Exercise Guidelines

The system in this book has been developed through my work with 50+ clients since 1992 and is part of the Nordic Body System. While it is a whole system, you can pull out segments and execute them individually. However, you will see the best results and success when you engage the whole system in its complete form.

Each month at Nordic Body, we change up the strength training workout. Within the month, you repeat nine strength training exercises. With an injury-free emphasis, you increase the intensity every week so by week four you are working out at maximum potential. By then, you are familiar with the exercises and you may also have modified them to fit your fitness level. At the end of the month, you can also see the progress you have made within the month. It's quite an incentive to keep going.

Then we reset in the first week of the next month, doing a whole new engaging workout at an easy intensity level, including low resistance. I vary the exercises and intensity with my clients so that they stay injury free as they are getting stronger.

Here's how you can use all the pieces you have explored within this book for the body, brain, and mind.

1. **Nordic Body Reboot Program:** If you have any ankle, knee, hip, or lower back aches and pains, I suggest you do the whole *Nordic Body Reboot Program* daily or every other day. It can either be part of a strength training workout or a cardiovascular workout or just by itself.

2. **Structure of a Nordic Body Strength Training Workout**
   a. **Warm- Up**
      i. Trigger Release
      ii. Dynamic Drill
      iii. 5 Warm-up repetitions prior to each first strength training exercise. (Does not apply to isometric ones since there is no movement. Instead start with an easier position like half plank prior to full plank.)
   b. **Workout**
      i. Strength Training 2-3 times a week. 1-3 sets, always going to fatigue with each exercise. Remember to vary it to decrease risks of injuries, boredom, and to always surprise the body in a good way.
      ii. Vary the intensity weekly to remain injury-free
         - Week 1 easy
         - Week 2 moderate
         - Week 3 moderate-heavy
         - Week 4 heavy
         - If there are 5 weeks in a month, return to moderate-heavy
      iii. Vary the exercises monthly
   c. **Static Stretching**

3. **Structure of a Nordic Body Cardiovascular Training Workout**

   a. **Warm- Up**

      i. Trigger Release

      ii. Dynamic Drill *Body Awareness*

      iii. Start Walking or Nordic Walking slowly and gradually increase the speed within 3-5 minutes.

   b. **Workout**

      i. Walking or Nordic Walking 3-5 times a week, 20-60 minutes at a moderate to vigorous intensity.

      ii. Remember to vary it to decrease risk of injuries, boredom, and to always surprise the body in a good way.

      - Vary route/program
      - Vary intensity and time
        - Continuous - same speed the whole time
        - Intervals - alternate speed from slow to fast
        - Vary terrains - hills, stairs, sand

   c. **Cool Down**

      i. Finish the last 2-5 minutes of Walking or Nordic Walking by gradually decreasing the speed

      ii. Static Stretching

4. **Active Resting Day**: Take 1 day off from working out, but not from leading an Active Lifestyle. Aim daily for 10,000 steps even on your "day off."

APPENDIX B

ADOPT-A-WALK

Adopt-A-Walk was created to make an active lifestyle more easily accessible within communities, improving the health of the people in a fun and easy way. As a health advocacy organization, we are committed to creating and promoting walking-friendly communities. We opened the very first Adopt-A-Walk loop in Santa Monica on June 29, 2019. Yay!

The number of gyms appear to grow as fast as the obesity crisis! That industry is clearly not serving or providing a healthy lifestyle for the people who need it the most. Adopt-A-Walk bridges the gap between the fitness industry and the community by offering alternatives with its specifically designed walking paths.

We team up with City Planners to decide the location of the permanent and specifically designed walking path. People living nearby the proposed path are encouraged to get involved in the creation of the path to increase the connection in the neighborhood.

The ideal length of an Adopt-A-Walk is one mile and the ideal layout is a loop. A specific sign indicates the start & finish and displays information about the walking path. Along the route are distance markers every 0.1mile, inspirational quotes, and leaning rails or natural places to rest. The permanently designated walking path becomes a natural meeting point for people wanting to go for a walk, meet new friends, and get to know their neighborhood. Do you want to add an Adopt-A-Walk loop in your neighborhood? Email us at healthy@adoptawalk.org and we will add it to our list as we move nationwide.

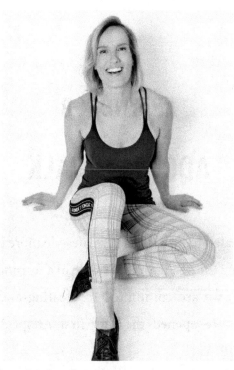

Originally from Sweden, Malin Svensson came to Los Angeles in 1989 with a master's degree in Physical Education. A former nationally ranked runner with over 30 years of experience in the fitness industry, Malin is the CEO & Founder of Nordic Body - a walking and fitness club committed to inspire the 50+ crowd to live a fun, healthy and fulfilling life by providing 360-degree support from **online** to **live programs** including **holistic fitness retreats**, **private sessions**, **workshops** and **community classes**.

Malin is also an **International Fitness Coach/Author/Speaker.** Whether she works out fitness guru **Jane Fonda** or people that have never worked out a day in their lives – her mission is the same: to strengthen the body and mind to age with confidence. Malin has been featured as a **walking and fitness expert** on CBS Los Angeles and in *LA Times*, *The NY Times*, *The Wall Street Journal* and *Fitness magazine*. She brought Nordic Walking to North America in 2002 and is one of the leading authorities in Nordic Walking worldwide. Her passion for making a difference in people's wellbeing is further expressed by her organization **Adopt-A-Walk**. The first 1-mile walking loop opened in Santa Monica on June 29, 2019.